RENEWING THE PROMISE

RENEWING THE PROMISE

Medicare and Its Reform

Edited by

David Blumenthal
Mark Schlesinger
Pamela Brown Drumheller

New York • Oxford
OXFORD UNIVERSITY PRESS
1988

Oxford University Press

Oxford New York Toronto
Delhi Bombay Calcutta Madras Karachi
Petaling Jaya Singapore Hong Kong Tokyo
Nairobi Dar es Salaam Cape Town
Melbourne Auckland

and associated companies in
Berlin Ibadan

Published by Oxford University Press, Inc.,
200 Madison Avenue, New York, New York 10016

Library of Congress Cataloging-in-Publication Data

Renewing the promise.

Includes background work and recommendations of the Harvard Medicare Reform Project.
Includes bibliographies and index.
1. Medicare—United States. I. Blumenthal, David, 1948– . II. Schlesinger, Mark. III. Drumheller, Pamela Brown. IV. Harvard Medicare Reform Project.
[DNLM: 1. Expenditures, Health—trends—United States.
2. Health Insurance for Aged and Disabled, Title 18.
WT 30 R411]
HD7102.U4M4283 1988 368.4'26'00973 87-24764
ISBN 0-19-504304-9

9 8 7 6 5 4 3 2 1

Printed in the United States of America
on acid-free paper

This book is dedicated to the memory of Wilbur R. Cohen: a happy warrior for compassionate and effective government, a principal parent of the Medicare program, and an inspiration to a generation of public servants who have seen government service as a noble calling.

Forward

At age twenty-three, the Medicare program is a remarkable governmental initiative. No program in the history of domestic federal legislation has done more to promote the health and well-being of America's elderly and disabled. Yet, for all its successes, the Medicare program is not without flaws, and there are reasons now for deep concern about its future.

Ongoing changes in the health care system—some of them hastened by Medicare—have rendered parts of its original design obsolete. Compromises deemed necessary to secure passage of the legislation in 1965 have come back to haunt the program in the form of escalating costs and confounding regulations.

At the same time, Medicare faces political challenges. In the drive to balance the federal budget, the program is a tempting target for cutbacks. In an era of governmental retrenchment, some propose doing away with Medicare entirely, replacing it with private medical retirement accounts or public subsidies for the elderly to purchase private insurance.

Participants in the Harvard Medicare Project saw the twentieth anniversary of this landmark initiative as an appropriate time to take stock of the challenges facing the Medicare program and to make specific suggestions for improvement. This volume is the product of two years of study and deliberation. It conveys the contributors' analysis of Medicare's accomplishments and failings, their assessment of alternative approaches to remedying those problems, the principles that guided their choice among options, and their recommendations for reform.*

In assimilating the product of their work, readers should be aware of several factors that helped to shape both their analysis and their recommendations. The contributors' approach to Medicare and its problems diverge in at least two important respects from some of the current political debate that swirls around Medicare in particular and health policy in general. First and foremost, the contributors have continually asked: How can the Medicare program be made better for its beneficiaries, for the elderly individuals who use and rely on it day in and day out? Members of the Harvard Medicare Project feel strongly that the current preoccupation with containing costs has become so overwhelming that relatively little attention is given to improving the program in ways that require few, if any, additional expenditures. As a result, valuable opportunities to improve the lives of our growing elderly population are being missed.

Second, although the contributors hope their findings will be relevant to issues now on the legislative agenda, as academics, they have the luxury of taking a longer

*Portions of this volume were previously published in David Blumenthal, Mark Schlesinger, Pamela Brown Drumheller et al. 1986: "The Future of Medicare." *New England Journal of Medicine* 314(11):722–28; and in Harvard Medicare Project, 1986, *Medicare: Coming of Age. A Proposal for Reform.* Boston: Division of Health Policy Research and Education, Harvard University. The Harvard Medicare Project.

view. In the past, Medicare reform has too often proceeded in a piecemeal manner, driven by moments of crisis or by purely programmatic concerns. This work takes a *comprehensive, long-term approach* to understanding Medicare's problems and to proposing change. Many of its suggestions indicate the direction the contributors think Medicare should take over the next 10 to 15 years. We hope history will bear them out and that this volume will contribute to a broad-ranging debate about the future of this essential but troubled program.

The volume itself consists of nine chapters. The first two review the history of Medicare legislation and the program's record to date, its accomplishments and its failings, in order to provide a background for the detailed examinations of outstanding policy issues that constitute the bulk of the rest of the book.

Chapter 3 confronts the first of these issues: whether the out-of-pocket costs borne by Medicare beneficiaries are appropriate in amount and fair in their distribution among elderly persons of differing incomes. Chapter 4 asks a somewhat different but closely related question: Does the Medicare program insure the elderly against the costs of the right kind of services in the right amounts to meet their changing health care needs?

Chapters 5 and 6 review Medicare's current methods for paying hospitals and physicians, whose services consume the great bulk of program expenditures. The authors of these two chapters consider possible approaches to the reimbursement of providers that might improve the program's fairness and efficiency. Chapter 7 considers the question of how Medicare should react to the challenges and opportunities posed by the development of innovative health care organizations, such as health maintenance organizations, preferred provider organizations, and life-care communities. How, if at all, should Medicare encourage or pay for the enrollment of beneficiaries in such organizations?

Chapter 8 reviews options for financing the Medicare program into the next century, and Chapter 9 presents the recommendations of the Harvard Medicare Project, which grew out of the background work represented in Chapters 1 through 8.

A great many individuals and organizations contributed to the work that made this volume possible. The Milbank Memorial Fund graciously funded the Harvard Medicare Project, whose findings have been previously reported and are summarized herein. The Richard King Mellon Foundation, through its generous support of the Harvard Division of Health Policy Research and Education, made possible the additional research and writing that culminated in this book. The Kennedy School of Government hosted the meetings, and a number of its faculty contributed selflessly to both the Project and this volume. We are particularly indebted to Hale Champion, who initially conceived the Project and guided it along the way.

Susan Hyde, Richard Minton, Kathleen Flynn and Alice Mullowney deserve special recognition for their tireless work in expediting the preparation of manuscripts. Barbara Gale and George Rosen helped in editing a number of chapters. We are grateful to Malka Kopell, Gail Meehan and Carol Cerf for their assistance in the early stages of the Project. Many people not listed as chapter authors also made important intellectual contributions to this volume, including Rashi Fein, Hale

Champion, Bob Binstock, Ted Marmor, Richard Margolis and the many scholars and health care policymakers who shared their views and comments with us during the preparation of *Medicare: Coming of Age, A Proposal for Reform*, the report of the Harvard Medicare Project.

Julius B. Richmond
David Blumenthal
Co-chairmen
Harvard Medicare Project

Contents

RENEWING THE PROMISE

1

Medicare: The Beginnings

DAVID BLUMENTHAL

. . . and every attempt
Is a wholly new start, and a different kind of failure
T. S. ELIOT, "EAST COKER"
Complete Poems, p. 128, V, ll 3–4.

The current state and future prospects of the Medicare program cannot be understood without a sense of the history of this momentous piece of social legislation. That history has been told a number of times, as befits one of the great federal initiatives of our time, the capstone of President Lyndon Johnson's Great Society (Feingold, 1966; Corning, 1969; Harris, 1969; Marmor, 1970; Feder, 1977; Cohen, 1985; David 1985). Yet, the story is worth telling again, if for no other reason than to temper with humility the ambitions of Medicare's latter-day reformers.

With the knowledge and certainty of hindsight, many students of Medicare have concluded, with some justification, that its current difficulties can be traced in large measure to provisions of the original legislation and the manner in which that legislation was implemented. If true, that observation should give us pause. For the Medicare program was crafted and enacted by experienced, some would even say brilliant, administrators and legislators after long years of struggle and debate. It was also enacted at a time of unique political opportunity when governmental institutions were simpler than they are today and when an electoral landslide had swept aside much of the opposition to federal health insurance for the elderly.

Could we have done better in their place? Can we do as well today? The answers to these questions are less important than the asking. One critical lesson of the history of the Medicare program is that even under the most favorable conditions, efforts at social reform are fraught with risks, both anticipated and unforeseen. By looking back at the events surrounding Medicare's early years, we may avoid repeating some past errors. But given the limits of our knowledge and the nature of our political institutions, new problems are inevitable. If nothing else, the history of this great social program teaches the need to design initiatives that are flexible and adaptable so that they can accommodate required reforms.

Subsequent chapters of this book will review in more detail the history of particular provisions of the Medicare program over the last twenty-three years. The remainder of this chapter recounts some of the key events before, during and immediately after the passage of the law, and highlights major forces that helped to shape the program's initial form and its development over time.

Legislative History

If the passage of federal legislation resembles a dance, as Redman (1973) contends, then the history of Medicare can be said to display almost every political step imaginable. Perhaps most astonishing is the way the tempo of events changed over time. The crafting of governmentally sponsored health insurance for the elderly proceeded for decades at such a slow and measured pace that progress was nearly indiscernible. In 1965, however, it climaxed in a flurry of legislative activity that produced in a matter of weeks the Medicare program as we know it today.

The Long Overture

The first legislation proposing federal health insurance for the elderly was introduced in 1952, but the history of Medicare really began in 1912 when Theodore Roosevelt, running for president on the Progressive party platform, first proposed the adoption of comprehensive national health insurance (NHI) (Corning, 1969; Harris, 1969). The ensuing debate over NHI progressed in fits and starts for 40 years. Faced with insurmountable political obstacles, the movement for NHI never really developed significant momentum, but the political storm it generated had a profound effect on the development and passage of Medicare.

In a strange historical anomaly, the American Medical Association (AMA) itself briefly supported the concept of NHI in 1916–17 (Harris, 1969), but a backlash from rural physicians and the laissez-faire political climate that was to prevail during the 1920s led to a permanent reversal in this position (Corning, 1969). The AMA assumed its now well-known stance as the nation's most vigorous opponent of governmentally sponsored health insurance in any form.

During the apparently properous and politically conservative 1920s, they had little to oppose because the idea of NHI went into dormancy. In Franklin Roosevelt's first term, the concept briefly resurfaced when, as part of the original Social Security legislation, the president proposed that the Social Security Board study the concept of federal health insurance. Faced with an avalanche of protesting telegrams from physicians, Roosevelt and the House Ways and Means Committee quickly dropped the idea for fear that the entire Social Security bill would go down in defeat (David, 1985).

This initial political outcome set the tone of the NHI debate for the next two decades. In 1939, Senator Robert F. Wagner, Sr. of New York introduced a bill that proposed matching federal grants to support state public health programs. Not a health insurance proposal as such, the bill nevertheless precipitated vigorous AMA opposition. After first backing the proposal, Roosevelt, who was running for reelection in 1940, withdrew his support at the last minute, and the Wagner bill died in committee. This victory contributed to what Harris (1969) has called the AMA's legend of invincibility, a reputation that was to dog proponents of federal involvement in health care.

Congressional advocates introduced a true NHI proposal in 1943, the Wagner-Murray-Dingell bill (named for its sponsors, Senator Wagner of New York, Senator James E. Murray of Montana, and Representative John D. Dingell of Michigan). After the 1944 election, Roosevelt is said to have been ready to support NHI, but with his death in 1945, health insurance again receded from the political agenda. It resurfaced, however, in January 1948 when President Harry Truman placed the full force of presidential advocacy behind the Wagner-Murray-Dingell bill in his State of the Union Address. It has been suggested that Truman's motives were as much tactical and political as anything else. He used Congress's refusal to act on NHI in his indictment of the "do-nothing" Congress, against which he successfully ran for reelection in 1948 (Harris, 1969). From the standpoint of NHI, however, his victory was largely Pyrrhic. His slim electoral margin and the continued hostility of the Congress, which was dominated by Republicans and conservative Southern Democrats, made the passage of NHI all but impossible (Corning, 1969).

The AMA did not share that view, however, and launched a now-legendary nationwide lobbying campaign aimed at killing NHI once and for all. Led by the public relations firm of Whittaker and Baxter, which had previously organized the successful defeat of a state health insurance plan in California, the campaign cost more than $4 million over the three years from 1948 to 1951. During that period, Whittaker and Baxter distributed tens of millions of posters, pamphlets and leaflets opposing NHI. A centerpiece of the effort was a poster reproducing a famous Luke Fildes painting. A physician, sitting head in hand, attends a sick little girl who lies asleep on pillows spread across two chairs. Helpless parents hover in the background. A caption reads, "Keep Politics Out of This Picture!" Copies appeared in thousands of doctors' offices around the United States.

On the advice of Whittaker and Baxter, the AMA had the personal physicians of members of Congress communicate their opposition to NHI directly to their influential patients. Perhaps most important, however, the public relations firm organized members of local medical societies to appear before nonmedical groups all over the country in search of endorsements for the AMA's position. Eventually, 1,829 such organizations officially supported the AMA in its struggle against NHI (Harris, 1969).

There was no progress on NHI during Truman's presidency, and in September 1952, the AMA declared victory in the battle to defeat NHI. The prominence of the AMA campaign, however, makes it easy to forget that other forces impeded the passage of health insurance. One of the most important of these was ideological. Partly as a result of AMA rhetoric, the debate over NHI, and later Medicare, became sharply polarized along ideological lines. Opponents of Medicare saw it as an attempt to increase the size and scope of governmental responsibilities and to redistribute resources between societal groups. Conservatives, then as today, opposed such policies on principle as dangerous intrusions on the freedoms of affected citizens. This explains the AMA's success in recruiting hundreds of other influential lobbying groups—from the Daughters of the American Revolution (DAR) to the U.S. Chamber of Commerce—to join in fighting NHI (Corning, 1969; Harris, 1969).

The ideological opposition to Medicare might not have been so potent if it were not for a second factor: the prevailing power structure of the Congress, whose key committees (especially House Ways and Means and Senate Finance) were dominated by conservative Southern Democrats and Northern Republicans during much of the postwar era. The composition of congressional committees was slow to change, and opponents of Medicare would later benefit significantly from the conservative tilt of these key House and Senate panels (Marmor, 1970).

By 1950, governmental advocates of federally sponsored health insurance had recognized the hopelessness of the NHI cause and began looking for a politically viable strategy for expanding protection against the cost of illness. The two men who had written the Wagner-Murray-Dingell-bill, Wilbur Cohen and I. S. Falk, were employed by the Federal Security Agency (FSA), which administered the Social Security program at the time. Thus, it was not by chance that they focused on health insurance for the elderly, the population group with which they were most familiar, as an alternative to a comprehensive plan. As Corning (1969) notes, "Social Security officials had been troubled by the fact that, as long as the social security system failed to protect against the single greatest cause of economic dependency in old age—the high cost of medical care—it could not really fulfill its basic objective" (p. 72).

In June 1951, Oscar Ewing, the head of FSA, first publicly proposed that, as part of their Social Security benefits, pensioners should receive 60 free days of hospital care. In April 1952, Senator Murray and Representative Dingell filed bills to this effect. Wilbur Cohen would later say:

> The new idea seemed pretty paltry at first—a trifling two hundred and thirty million dollars a year. In the beginning, we looked at it as a small way to start something big—what the AMA would call a "foot in the door." But in time the bill we wrote—or, anyway, the idea behind it—became our *only* goal. . . . Anyway, it's all been very Hegelian. The state and federal proposals for compulsory health insurance were the thesis, the AMA's violent opposition was the antithesis, and Medicare is the synthesis (Harris, 1969, p. 55).

The Quickening Pace

Despite Cohen's cheerful tone, there is no question that the long confrontation with the AMA and other conservatives had fundamentally altered the terms of the Medicare debate. Advocates of NHI were on the political defensive, and they embraced the cause of health insurance for the elderly in large measure because of its political appeal. Indeed, throughout the campaign to pass an elderly health care bill, proponents seemed to weigh political factors as heavily as substantive issues in crafting the program's details. As Marmor (1970, p. 23) has noted, they adopted the tactic of "concensus mongering: the identification of less-disputed problems and the advocacy of modest solutions." One example of this was the explicit decision of Medicare's crafters and their congressional allies to focus on hospital and nursing home benefits and to drop physician coverage for the elderly in the hopes that this would make the program less offensive to key committee chairpersons (Feingold, 1966).

From a political standpoint, the decision to focus on health insurance for the elderly was inspired. The elderly go to the polls, and even in the 1950s, demographic trends made clear that they were growing rapidly in numbers. As a defined group with certain common interests (not the least of which was their need for health insurance), they were also easier to organize and mobilize than the electorate as a whole. If politicians opposed health care for the elderly, they ran the risk of seeming to be against aged Americans.

The circumstances of elderly Americans in the 1950s also undercut some of the ideological and practical objections of conservatives to NHI. Conservatives opposed universal NHI, at least in part, because it would involve the government in dispensing benefits to individuals who did not really need such assistance, who could afford to pay for health care or health insurance on their own. As a group, however, the elderly were far more needy of governmental assistance than the typical American. In the 1950s, the elderly were clearly less affluent than the average American. Thirty-five percent of elders in 1959 were poor as compared with 22 percent of the country as a whole (Gornick et al., 1985). A 1962 study from the University of Michigan showed that the health care expenses of the aged were more than twice those of younger Americans (Feingold, 1966), yet many lacked health care insurance. Though the AMA and health insurers claimed in the early 1960s that 50 to 53 percent of the elderly had health insurance, a Senate investigation indicated that only half that many elderly had meaningful protection against the costs of hospitalization (Corning, 1969; Harris, 1969). Policies typically covered only one quarter of the hospital expenses of elders who were insured. Other studies showed that the elderly who rated their health as poor were only half as likely to have insurance as those who rated their health as good. Even the Eisenhower administration admitted the health care problems of the elderly were severe. In a 1959 report to the Ways and Means Committee, the Department of Health, Education and Welfare (DHEW—now the Department of Health and Human Services [DHHS]) noted:

> Older persons have larger than average medical care needs. As a group they use about two-and-a-half times as much general hospital care as the average for persons under the age of 65. . . . Their incomes are generally considerably lower than those of the rest of the population. . . . Because both the number and proportion of older persons in the population are increasing, a satisfactory solution to the problem of paying for adequate medical care for the aged will become more rather than less important (Corning, 1969, p. 81).

Conservatives further opposed NHI and other governmental aid programs for the poor and nonpoor on the grounds that they undermined incentives for recipients to work and provide for themselves. As Marmor (1970) points out, advocates of health insurance for the elderly sought to neutralize that argument by tying the program to the Social Security system. Social Security beneficiaries received no benefits unless they made the requisite payments during their working years. A health insurance program provided on the same terms and through the same mechanism, therefore, would not undermine the work ethic. To put the point somewhat differently, elderly recipients of health care benefits funded by Social Security payments were inherently deserving of those benefits because they had already paid for them through decades of Social Security contributions.

Linking health care for the elderly to Social Security had another advantage for proponents of elderly health insurance. It associated the new health care benefit with a popular and highly legitimate public program. Part of that legitimacy, advocates felt, derived from the fact that the program was universal: All workers contributed and all received benefits, regardless of income.

Many conservatives felt that any new health insurance benefit for the elderly should be means tested, that is, related in some way to the recipients' ability to pay. Conservatives felt that this was the only way to ensure that beneficiaries were truly needy, as even among the elderly there were many individuals with the resources to purchase their own insurance or pay for their own care. Advocates of health insurance strongly disagreed. They feared that means testing a health insurance program would associate it with politically vulnerable welfare programs in the minds of the aged and the electorate as a whole. As a universal program of social insurance, Social Security did not involve means testing. By incorporating a health insurance benefit into the package of benefits provided by Social Security, proponents hoped Medicare could avoid the requirement to relate eligibility or benefits to the income of recipients and escape the stigma attached to governmental welfare initiatives.

Though aware of these political advantages to their revised strategy, proponents of NHI were also acutely aware that they still faced formidable opposition from members of key congressional committees and outside lobby groups. They took pains, therefore, to design a program that would be as difficult as possible for antagonists to oppose.

First and foremost, they proposed an almost irreducible minimum of benefits. This is exemplified by Oscar Ewing's initial proposal that Social Security cover only 60 days of hospital care. Somewhat expanded benefit packages were contained in later bills introduced in 1957 by Representative Aime Forand of Rhode Island, and in 1961 by Representative Cecil King of California and Senator Clinton Anderson of New Mexico. These later bills, however, were still far from comprehensive. The King-Anderson bill represented official policy during both the Kennedy and Johnson administrations. It covered 90 days of hospital care, 180 days of nursing home care, outpatient diagnostic services, and 240 home visits by a nurse. In a vain effort to deflect AMA opposition, the King-Anderson bill provided no coverage for physician services, unlike the Forand bill, which at least insured the elderly against the cost of inpatient surgical fees.

In a further effort to reassure provider groups, the King-Anderson bill offered assurances that nothing in the legislation should be construed to give federal agencies the authority to alter the practice of medicine, the provision of hospital or nursing home care, or the management of hospital or nursing home personnel (Harris, 1969).

Despite these tactical adjustments, little happened for about six years after health care for the elderly was first proposed. Toward the end of the 1950s, however, the efforts of Medicare proponents began to pay off. Elderly groups, organized with the assistance of the American Federation of Labor and Congress of Industrial Organizations (AFL–CIO), began speaking out and pressuring congressmen and senators. In 1958, the House Ways and Means Committee held hearings on health insurance for the elderly for the first time. In 1959, the Senate created the Subcommittee on Problems of the Aged and Aging, and it discovered strong sentiment for health insurance protection among aged witnesses in regional hearings (David, 1985).

Perhaps most important, John F. Kennedy increasingly made health insurance for the elderly an issue in his campaign for the presidency (David, 1985). Recognizing the political power of this issue and contemplating his own candidacy, Vice President Nixon began pleading with reluctant Republican leaders to formulate a

Republican position on health care for the elderly. In the spring of 1960, Nixon prevailed on the administration to introduce a Medicare program of its own, one that would have subsidized state programs to help the elderly purchase limited private health insurance plans (Harris, 1969).

Neither the Democrat's Forand bill nor the Republican proposal had much support in the House Ways and Means Committee, but Wilbur Mills (Democrat from Arkansas), the committee's savvy chairman, could recognize a preelection political stampede when he stood in its path. In April 1960, Walter Reuther, head of the United Auto Workers (UAW) and a strong proponent of Medicare, prevailed on Sam Rayburn and John McCormack, Democratic leaders of the House of Representatives, to meet with Mills and urge his support for an elderly health insurance program linked to Social Security. Eventually, Rayburn, Lyndon Johnson (then Senate Majority Leader and an aspiring presidential candidate) and Reuther met with Mills, who agreed to report an elderly health care bill (David, 1985). Instead of the Forand bill, however, he rapidly introduced and shepherded through his committee and the House of Representatives a health care program that he could live with—an expansion of the existing Old Age Assistance program that, since 1956, had provided limited funds to states to cover the health care costs of the very poor elderly. Comparable legislation quickly passed the Senate under the sponsorship of a powerful conservative member of the Senate Finance Committee, Democrat Robert Kerr of Oklahoma. Known as the Kerr-Mills bill, this new legislation allowed for unlimited federal support of health care for needy elderly but only so long as states provided matching funds. It left to the states the job of defining standards of need and levels of benefit. As a means-tested, welfare program administered at the state level, it was far more acceptable to conservatives than a universal health insurance program for the aged funded through Social Security and administered by the federal government.

Thus, after eight years, the new strategy of focusing on health care for the elderly had produced its first results. Though not what Cohen, Falk, Ewing, and their allies had wanted, they were not entirely displeased with the Kerr-Mills bill. Cohen had actually written the Senate version of the legislation at Kerr's request. Cohen's motives were tactical. He felt that providing health care to the nation's very needy elderly had value in itself and that a broader program could be added on top of it. He felt that so few states would cooperate that the welfare approach would be widely criticized, thus opening the field to a program funded and administered through Social Security. He also sought to win the trust of members of the key congressional committees by demonstrating that he was willing to provide dispassionate technical assistance even for legislation with which he disagreed (Conversation with Wilbur J. Cohen at John F. Kennedy School of Government in Cambridge, Massachusetts, on March 8, 1974, as well as a written communication from him on November 7, 1986).

Shared by other Medicare proponents inside and outside the Congress, Cohen's prediction that Kerr-Mills would fail to meet the needs of elderly Americans was quickly vindicated. By 1963, only 32 of the 50 states had undertaken health care initiatives under Kerr-Mills, and 88 percent of federal funds were going to 5 states with particularly active programs: California, Massachusetts, Michigan, New York, and Pennsylvania (David, 1985). In the meantime, labor unions, the elderly, and a new Democratic administration intensified their advocacy of universal health insurance for the aged.

In his first State of the Union Address, President Kennedy renewed his commitment to broadened health insurance for retirees. Wilbur Cohen became assistant secretary for legislation in DHEW. Aware that he lacked the votes in the House Ways and Means Committee to pass the King-Anderson bill, Kennedy worked with the Democratic House leadership to alter the composition of the committee. To increase popular pressure on the Congress the Democratic National Committee and the AFL–CIO continued their efforts to organize the elderly by creating the National Council of Senior Citizens, which was led by Congressman Forand, who had just retired (Corning, 1969). In May 1962, the Kennedy administration organized 33 rallies around the country in which leading members of the administration spoke on behalf of Medicare. Kennedy himself spoke at a nationally televised rally in New York's Madison Square Garden. Then, in July 1962, the president pushed the King-Anderson bill to a vote in the Senate, losing by a narrow 52-to-48 margin (Corning, 1969).

Meanwhile, the AMA suffered a self-inflicted defeat when it organized the American Medical Political Action Committee (AMPAC) in 1961 and tried to defeat pro-Medicare congressmen in the 1962 election. The AMA campaign had little effect. As Sundquist (1968, p. 314) notes, "The people's verdict was for medicare. . . . Organized medicine could not claim to have been instrumental in defeating a single pro-medicare senator or congressman. On the contrary, enough new Democrats were elected to the Senate to reverse that body's 1962 decision. Six Democrats, all supporters of medicare, defeated six Republican opponents of the measure."

After Kennedy's death, Lyndon Johnson proved every bit as committed to Medicare as the slain president, and he pursued the goal with his legendary political skills. Facing the 1964 congressional election, under pressure from Johnson and the Democratic leadership in the House to report the King-Anderson bill, the Ways and Means Committee considered Medicare in closed executive session from March to June. Eventually, the committee defeated the bill by one vote, but the Senate forced the issue by passing King-Anderson on September 2, 1964. Barry Goldwater, Republican of Arizona and Republican nominee for the presidency, made a dramatic return from the campaign trail to vote against the legislation (Sundquist, 1968). A hotly contested conference ensued that dragged on for over a month and adjourned in deadlock after Mills refused to accept King-Anderson as an amendment to pending Social Security legislation. Though consistent with past positions, Mills's intransigence probably reflected the feelings of the average House member, for whom a vote either way on Medicare was bound to offend an important constituency in the upcoming election (Harris, 1969).

Doubletime

In the 1964 election, 22 percent of the vote was cast by citizens over the age of 60. As if that were not enough to demonstrate the power of the Medicare constituency, Lyndon Johnson was returned to office with a huge personal mandate, and a two-to-one Democratic majority in the House. Both Goldwater and Johnson had made Medicare a major issue in their respective campaigns, as had many members of Congress. The popular verdict seemed clear. "The 1964 Democratic landslide settled the issue," notes Sundquist (1968, p. 317). "Practically the entire Democratic 'class of '64' in the House . . . was committed to Medicare."

To reflect the House's new composition, the membership of the House Ways and Means Committee was changed from 15 Democrats and 10 Republicans to 17 Democrats and 8 Republicans. In January 1965, Johnson sent a special health message to the Congress again urging passage of the King-Anderson bill, which, as the first bill filed during the Eighty-ninth session of the Congress, was now called H.R. 1. Ever the realist, Mills publicly committed himself to reporting some form of health care bill for the elderly by March.

After 53 years of wrangling over federal provision of health care insurance, events now began to accelerate. In moves that would have major, unforeseen consequences, the AMA and the Republicans shifted their positions on Medicare in order to control the damage done by the 1964 elections.

To begin with, the AMA sought to counter support for King-Anderson by pointing out, paradoxically, that its benefits were too limited. In its place, they offered their own program, Eldercare, which would empower the federal government to fund state programs that subsidized more comprehensive private health insurance programs (including coverage of physicians' services) for the elderly. For their part, the Republicans focused their strongest attack on the fact that H.R. 1 was compulsory. They proposed a federally administered but voluntary program of comprehensive health insurance that, like Eldercare, would cover physicians' services but, unlike alternative proposals, would be financed in part by beneficiary premiums and in part by general revenues. Introduced by Representative John Byrnes of Wisconsin, ranking Republican on the House Ways and Means Committee, the bill was modeled on private policies offered by the Aetna Insurance Company. Mills took the House Ways and Means Committee into executive session in January 1965, where six weeks of intense but inconclusive discussion ensured. Then, on March 2, Wilbur Mills made a suggestion that had profound consequences for American health care. Without warning, he asked Wilbur Cohen, who was present to provide technical assistance, whether compulsory hospital insurance of the sort proposed under H.R. 1 could be combined with a voluntary program of physicians' insurance similar to the Byrnes proposal. Further, he asked whether a third component—an expanded version of the Kerr-Mills bill—covering the health care expenditures of all poor Americans could be added. Mills himself had introduced this Medicaid precursor in January.

Cohen describes what happened next:

> I answered that it was possible. I had no specific authority from anyone to underwrite such a proposal, but I had enough common sense not to dismiss it out of hand. . . . Mills did not spell out any specifics to me. Rather, he urged prompt action on a draft of such a proposal. I asked for a little more time to complete such a major undertaking. Mills said no, he wanted it the next day. I felt he sensed he had caught the critics off guard, and he did not want them to have time to regroup. He was like a general who saw he could rout his opposition and follow them as they retreated. . . . It was a brilliant tour de force (Cohen, 1985, p. 6).

In comments to Harris, Cohen described the political rationale behind Mills's masterstroke. By expanding the benefits of Medicare to include physicians' services, Mills met the AMA criticism that King-Anderson was too narrow. By incorporating the Byrnes proposal, he gave the Republicans recognition and a stake in supporting the bill. He also made physicians' coverage voluntary rather than compulsory, which would meet the objections of opponents to mandatory participation in the program, at least for some part of its provisions. "Mills had taken the AMA's ammunition, put it in the Republican's gun, and blown both of them off the map," Cohen chuckled (Harris, 1969, p. 187).

After his exchange with Cohen, Mills promptly adjourned the committee, scheduling a meeting for the next day. Leaving Robert Ball, commissioner of Social Security, in charge of drafting, Cohen dashed back to his office and

> fortunately, found President Johnson in the nearby office occupied by John Gardner, the Secretary of HEW. I barged in and briefly told the President what had occurred. . . . The President did not bat an eye. He accepted the situation calmly, which I took for approval and clearance. It was a strange and unique way in which to make a major policy decision. There was no policy clearance with others in the Department or in the Budget Bureau or White House. Mills had scored a coup. Johnson immediately realized it. I was the intermediary for a major expansion of our proposal without any intervening review of the details of the proposal as developed by the staff. In this case, the Federal Government was moving into a major area of medical care with practically no review of alternatives, options, trade-offs or costs (Cohen, 1985, p. 6).

Marmor faults the administration for being so totally unprepared for Mills's expanded Medicare proposal, "The long process of building support for a hospitalization program covering the aged had not prepared the Johnson Administration for the unpredictable opportunities of 1965," he notes (Marmor, 1970, p. 81). However, given the end run that Mills (with Cohen's willing support) had engineered around the bureaucratic policy process, it is not clear that elaborate staff work would have mattered. Indeed, one senses that Mills's haste was intended as much to avoid bureaucratic and political entanglements in the executive branch as to keep the AMA and the Republicans on the defensive. After all, some Democratic constituency groups had long opposed voluntary federal health insurance programs like the new proposed Part B of Medicare.

Puzzling as it may seem, Mills's own personal conversion from opponent to architect of reform reflected numerous motivations. In the narrowest sense, as a consummate political tactician, he recognized the inevitability of Medicare and wanted to be able to take credit for its passage.

On another level, however, he sought control over the process in order to achieve certain policy goals of his own. Mills considered the protection of the Social Security system and the solvency of its trust fund as one of his primary missions as chairman of the House Ways and Means Committee. "The first responsibility of the Committee on Ways and Means and, indeed, the entire Congress, to this system of social insurance," Mills told a Little Rock, Arkansas, audience in September 1964, "is to see that it is maintained on a sound financial basis" (Mills, 1964, p. 24015). He felt a "deep concern," he told his constituents, that universal health insurance for the elderly, if financed through Social Security, could threaten its financial integrity (Mills, 1964, p. 24016). Mills further recognized that the benefits under King-Anderson were inadequate and that after its passage the elderly might be bitterly disappointed (Starr, 1982). The pressure to include physicians' services might then become irresistible. Therefore, Mills embraced a voluntary Part B that would be funded largely through general revenues. He viewed this as a way to avoid future pressures to expand the part of Medicare that was to be funded through Social Security. As further protection for the fiscal integrity of the original Social Security trust fund, he also created a wholly separate trust fund within Social Security to pay for Medicare hospital benefits.

In broadening Medicare and especially in adding Medicaid to the package, Mills also sought to forestall a development that some of Medicare's advocates fervently sought: the creation of a national health insurance program. Cohen (1985, p. 3) recalls an exchange with Mills during the Medicare debate:

> The inclusion of Medicaid in the 1965 law evolved when Mr. Wilbur Mills asked me what his answer should be to the inevitable question he thought he would be asked during the legislative debate: "Isn't Medicare an 'entering wedge' to a broader program of nationwide 'compulsory' insurance for everyone?" I suggested that if he included some plan to cover the key groups of poor people he would have a possible answer to this criticism. Medicaid evolved from this problem and discussion. I developed most of the provisions by expanding the plan requirements in the Kerr-Mills bill of 1960.

The events of March 3, 1965, proved almost anticlimactic. Cohen presented a draft of the legislative "three-layer cake" that Mills had proposed. Mills said, "OK, it sounds fine" (Harris, 1969, p. 188). Though the committee continued to discuss the bill in executive session for almost a month thereafter, the outcome was never in doubt. With the chairman on board and with the revised committee membership, the vote was a foregone conclusion. The Republicans offered numerous amendments, but all were beaten back. Democratic committee members yielded to Mills's greater expertise (David, 1985). Though Republicans on Ways and Means voted against it en bloc, the committee approved Medicare on March 23, and the full House passed it two weeks later.

One reason that Mills's footwork was so successful may have been that the bill approved by the committee still contained a number of sweeteners for providers that were viewed as essential to its passage and implementation. These included Section 1801 of Title XVIII, which was held over from the King-Anderson bill:

> Nothing in this title shall be construed to authorize any Federal officer or employee to exercise any supervision or control over the practice of medicine or the manner in which medical services are provided, or over the selection, tenure, or compensation of any officer or employee of any institution, agency, or person providing health services; or to exercise any supervision or control over the administration or operation of any such institution, agency or person.

In other words, the federal government would continue to keep its hands off the practice of medicine and provision of institutional health care services. To reinforce this assurance, Parts A and B were to be administered by intermediaries and carriers, respectively, which were to be private health insurance companies. Because providers were generally comfortable with their treatment at the hands of such private companies, this was intended to reassure them that the federal government, insofar as possible, would confine its work to collecting taxes and channeling revenues to doctors and hospitals. Hospitals were even permitted to pick the intermediary they wanted to deal with (Thompson, 1981). The House-approved legislation also retained the King-Anderson bill's provision that hospitals were to be paid "reasonable costs" for their services as well as Byrnes bill's provisions that physicians were to be paid their "reasonable and customary" fees, a stipulation modeled on existing Blue Shield and Aetna practices. Consistent with the precursor bills for Parts A and B and with existing private plans, both sections of the legislation retained deductible and coinsurance provisions designed to reduce federal costs and deter unnecessary utilization.

Though they occasioned some discussion, none of these issues, with the exception of the bill's coinsurance and deductible provisions, became the objects of major debate in the Senate or in conference between the Senate and the House. Prompt Senate consideration of the legislation was assured through one of Lyndon Johnson's celebrated political maneuvers. Three days after the House Ways and Means Committee passed its version of Medicare, Johnson went on national television with nine congressional Democratic leaders to hail the bill's passage. Among those present was Harry F. Byrd, Democrat of Virginia, chairman of the Senate Finance Committee, and no friend of federal health insurance legislation. In an amusing exchange detailed by Johnson (1971) in his memoirs, the president first got a reluctant Byrd to admit before millions of viewers that the Finance Committee had no pressing business that would preclude consideration of Medicare and then persuaded him to hold prompt hearings on the bill.

In the ensuing consideration of the legislation, senators did raise some issues with long-term significance for the program. Senator Russell Long, Democrat of Louisiana, (who replaced Byrd as chairman of Senate Finance in the middle of the bill's debate) played a pivotal role in Medicare's brief but intense passage through the Senate. Taking a position reminiscent of the AMA's view of King-Anderson, Long attacked the House-passed version as offering inadequate benefits—in this case, insufficient protection against the costs of catastrophic illness. He offered an amendment in committee that would make Medicare's hospital and physician benefits unlimited and finance the additional costs through a sliding scale of coinsurance and deductibles related to the patient's ability to pay. Thus, in one deft stroke, Long highlighted both a real deficiency in the program, its limited coverage of costs, and a political and ethical problem that would later trouble Medicare's proponents as well as its opponents: The wealthy elderly benefited as much or more than the very poor elderly from Medicare.

Though apparently intended to give the elderly better coverage, Long's amendment was widely viewed by Medicare's advocates as an attempt to make the legislation so expensive that the House would reject it completely (Harris, 1969). Thus, for short-term political purposes, liberals coalesced to force Long to drop catastrophic coverage, which in later years many would admit was badly needed. To win over some supporters of broader hospital coverage, such as Democratic Senator Abraham Ribicoff of Connecticut, the bill's proponents agreed to add 60 days of hospital coverage (with a $10-a-day coinsurance fee) to the original 60 free days provided by the House bill (after a $40 deductible). The proposal for means-tested coinsurance and deductibles was beaten back. Thus, the bill's benefits were reluctantly expanded by liberals in order to defeat a perceived conservative challenge.

The Senate generally exerts less discipline over its members than the House during floor debate, but this was not the only reason that more than five hundred amendments were added to the Medicare bill before it was passed on July 9. As floor manager and majority whip, Long made no effort to prevent amendments, even those proposing changes that had been defeated in committee. Clinton Anderson, for one, interpreted Long's behavior as a further attempt to frustrate passage of the legislation and to complicate the House-Senate conference (Harris, 1969). As a result, the Senate again had to beat back an amendment that would have made hospital benefits unlimited under Part A.

By the time it had passed the two houses of the U.S. Congress, Medicare (with Medicaid quietly in tow) was not one three-layer cake, but two. In conference, the two versions were pieced together to make a single but more complex whole. One of Mills's goals was to reduce the scope of the more expensive Senate bill. House-Senate conferees picked and chose among contrasting provisions, frequently retaining deductibles or coinsurance where one body had them but the other did not. On some key provisions, such as extent of hospital coverage, the conferees split the difference, compromising midway between House and Senate bills. Only one relatively minor issue provoked sharp controversy. At Mills's insistence, the House bill had permitted hospital-based physicians (pathologists, radiologists, anesthesiologists and psychiatrists) to bill Medicare independently under Part B. The Senate had rejected this provision. Critics of Mills's approach viewed it as an invitation for these physicians, who in the past had generally worked on salary, to charge high fees at the government's expense. Mills, however, viewed this provision as part of a promise he had made not to intrude on the way physicians and hospitals organized their business. Despite strong pressure from the White House on down, Mills prevailed.

In late July, after both houses of Congress had considered the revised bill reported by their conferees, Medicare and Medicaid were passed into law. The legislation was promptly signed by President Johnson at a ceremony in Independence, Missouri, in the presence of former president Harry Truman, during whose term Oscar Ewing first proposed federal health insurance for the elderly.

The End of the Beginning

When the music stopped, participants in the Medicare dance found themselves in unanticipated postures. Long-term enemies of national health insurance had dramatically expanded Medicare's benefits. Long-term advocates of federal health care insurance were opposing efforts to increase coverage. Both sides were preoccupied with their own political nightmares: Conservatives tried to prevent the creation of true NHI or to slow Medicare by overstuffing it; liberals tried to keep the bill lean enough so that it wouldn't topple into still another legislative defeat.

The product of the legislative dance was unanticipated as well. Medicare emerged as a broader, more generous health care program than even its most fervent supporters had thought possible. But it also emerged containing the seeds of future, unforeseen problems. These problems would not be easily rectified, for their origins were deeply rooted in the history and politics of this great health care initiative and the legislative process that produced it.

Paying the Piper

The first and most widely cited deficiency in the original Medicare law was the way in which its payment policies encouraged the escalation of health care costs. The details concerning Medicare's explosive expenditures are explored subsequently, especially in Chapters 5 and 6, which deal with issues of provider payment. For now, we note only that by paying hospitals on the basis of reasonable costs and physicians on the basis of usual and customary fees, Medicare has undoubtedly contributed to the rapid increases in health care expenditures that have bedeviled the program itself and the health care system generally.

Commenting on the provision to pay hospitals "reasonable costs," Cohen has made the following point:

> The principle . . . was never seriously debated or opposed during the period 1961–65, as far as I can recollect. . . . No one thought of it as a basis for inflationary price or cost rises. It was accepted not only because no other alternative was proposed, but because conventional wisdom at the time accepted reasonable cost as a reasonable principle. (Cohen, 1985, p. 8)

The same circumstances undoubtedly shaped the choice of payment policies for physicians. In its approach to compensating physicians and hospitals, Congress was copying existing private plans that provided the only precedent on how to proceed. "There was only a limited amount of experience with large-scale, nationwide, health reimbursement programs," Cohen (1985, p. 3) recalls. "There was a good deal of rhetoric and little empirical information."

Even if such information had existed, it is not clear that Congress would or could have acted differently. As Cohen himself has noted, Mills, with Cohen's acquiescence, pushed through the House version of Medicare with such haste that thorough review of its cost (or other) consequences was impossible. Mills's decision to proceed in this fashion reflected short-term political considerations: a desire to throw opponents off balance so that he could shape a program that was both politically viable and consistent with his programmatic goals.

More fundamental political issues, however, were also at work in shaping Congress's approach to paying hospitals and physicians. The long history of vehement provider resistance had convinced supporters and opponents of federal health insurance for the elderly that unless legislation paid providers the way they wanted to be paid, they would refuse to see Medicare patients. Indeed, even paying generously might not be enough. At an AMA convention on June 20, 1965, nine state delegations introduced resolutions favoring a boycott of the pending Medicare law.

The fear of provider revolt and a well-developed respect for their congressional influence help to explain why advocates of King-Anderson were unprepared to react to Mills's proposal to incorporate Part B into Medicare and why there was so little consideration of alternative payment schemes. Irwin Wolkstein (1970, p. 699), who worked with Cohen, Ball and others in crafting the Medicare legislation, has noted:

> Some might think that all the . . . concessions made to the insurance and health establishment were unnecessary from a political point of view in 1965 since at

> that time the House of Representatives, following the Democratic landslide victory in the election of 1964, was composed of the highest proportion of liberal legislators in many years. Yet the key vote on Medicare in the House in 1965 carried by a margin of just forty-five votes. . . . The opposition to the bill was based in significant part on concern about the degree of federal invasion into medical care that would result.

As Feder (1977) has documented, concern about provider opposition also dominated initial implementation of the Medicare legislation. Officials at the Social Security Agency (SSA)—which administered Medicare until the Health Care Financing Administration (HCFA) was created in 1977—sought above all to assure that providers would be there when elderly patients sought their services. "The primary objective of 1965–67," Cohen (1985, p. 8) recalls, "was to get off to a good start, to avoid any strike, slowdown, or other uncooperative action."

Administrators in Social Security initially took a fairly tough stance in negotiating reimbursement formulae for the operating and capital costs of hospitals. However, facing strong opposition from the American Hospital Association (AHA) and the need to get agreement by July 1, 1966, officials in SSA and DHEW backed down and agreed to a much more generous payment formula that included the now infamous 2-percent-plus factor. For the first few years after Medicare was enacted, the program paid hospitals 2 percent more than their identifiable allowable costs in order to permit them to replace capital stock as it depreciated (Thompson, 1981). "Where they had discretion," Feder (1977, p. 69) notes, "administrators consciously subordinated fiscal control to hospital cooperation, thereby fueling the inflation they had tried to avoid."

Once established, this attitude toward program administration would prove very hard to change; indeed, the system offered few political incentives to take a much tougher stance with providers. Although Congress, especially the Senate Finance Committee, frequently criticized SSA reimbursement formulae as inflationary, it often diluted or rejected stringent proposals for reform. In 1970, for example, SSA proposed for the first time that hospitals be prospectively paid for caring for Medicare patients. Congress reacted by authorizing experiments with such payment schemes (Feder, 1977; Thompson, 1981). It took 13 years of experimentation before Congress acted on this idea in 1983, adopting, ironically, a prospective payment system (PPS) that had been tried but never evaluated.

Congress and SSA were not alone in lacking the stomach or the knowledge to design payment schemes that might encourage prudence or restraint in the provision of services. Private insurers and corporations treated the health professions with comparable generosity for nearly two decades after Medicare was passed (Califano, 1986). As Starr (1982) has pointed out, Congress's approach to paying providers under Medicare seems to have reflected a broadly shared social consensus that favored "redistribution without reorganization," that sought to make health care available to the elderly and the poor without making the tough structural changes necessary to control costs. It would take many years of dizzying health care inflation and many unsuccessful halfway attempts at reform before the American people and their government would be ready to make the difficult reforms in provider reimbursement that they avoided in 1965 (Brown, 1985).

Limits on Benefits

Despite its generous treatment of physicians and hospitals, it would be wrong to say that Congress was totally unconcerned about health care costs during the Medicare debate. In fact, the subject came up repeatedly but almost always in the context of deciding what benefits Medicare should cover and how much it should require consumers to pay out-of-pocket. When Congress wanted to reduce potential program costs, it reduced the number of covered hospital days, nursing home days, or home health care visits or it added deductibles for physicians' services and coinsurance for extended hospital stays.

Given the ideological and political history of the Medicare debate, this approach is not surprising. Conservatives had all along opposed universal compulsory federal health insurance. They feared its benefits would be abused by patients who did not really need or deserve federal assistance, either because they weren't ill or had the private means to purchase their own care. For their part, liberals, after the final defeat of NHI in 1950, had sought to make their Medicare proposal more acceptable to conservatives and the professions by reducing the proposed benefits to the minimum they, the health insurance advocates, could live with. Thus, when the election of 1964 opened the door of political opportunity, none of the central actors involved in Medicare saw the expansion of benefits as a critical goal. Only because of Mills's desire to protect the Social Security program and to preempt more comprehensive future legislation did Medicare emerge in the expanded form it assumed.

Evans (1985) and others have argued that it would have been possible to expand Medicare's benefits and contain the program's costs if its architects had been willing to restrict provider incomes, that is, reimbursement. We will never know if that would have proved the case. The approach Congress adopted implicitly assumed that any fiscal problems would result from consumer rather than provider abuse of the system. As we will see, one result was that Medicare had gaps in coverage that greatly increased the program's complexity, added to beneficiaries' confusion and required continuing out-of-pocket expenditures for a sizable fraction of elderly Americans.

In retrospect, therefore, Medicare's needlessly complex structure, limited benefits and overly generous provider-payment policies, can be attributed at least in part to the influence of a variety of political and legislative factors that had their roots in a long and continuing debate over national health insurance and the role of the federal government in providing health care to the American people. Perhaps Medicare's crafters could have done better in anticipating and preventing these problems; perhaps not. Medicare's legislative history provides valuable insight into the difficulties of social reform in the health care field. That history, however, provides inspiration as well. For, as we will see, the accomplishments of this extraordinary federal initiative have been every bit as remarkable as its failings.

REFERENCES

Brown, Lawrence D. 1985. Technocratic Corporation and Administrative Reform in Medicare. *Journal of Health Politics, Policy and Law* 10 (3):579–99.

Califano, Joseph A. 1986. *The American Health Care Revolution: Who Lives? Who Dies? Who Pays?* New York: Random House.

Cohen, Wilbur J. 1985. Reflections on the Enactment of Medicare and Medicaid. *Health Care Financing Review, 1985 Annual Supplement*, pp. 3–11.

Corning, Peter A. 1969. *The Evolution of Medicare . . . from Idea to Law*. U.S. Department of Health, Education and Welfare.

David, Sheri I. 1985. *With Dignity. The Search for Medicare and Medicaid.* Westport, CT: Greenwood Press.

Evans, Robert G. 1985. Illusions of Necessity: Evading Responsibility for a Choice in Health Care. *Journal of Health Politics, Policy and Law* 10 (3):439–67.

Feder, Judith M. 1977. *Medicare: The Politics of Federal Hospital Insurance.* Lexington, MA: Lexington Books.

Feingold, Eugene. 1966. *Medicare: Policy and Politics.* San Francisco: Chandler.

Gornick, Marian, Jay N. Greenberg, Paul W. Eggers et al., 1985. Twenty Years of Medicare and Medicaid: Covered Populations, Use of Benefits, and Program Expenditures. *Health Care Financing Review, 1985 Annual Supplement*, pp. 13–59.

Harris, Richard. 1969. *A Sacred Trust*. Baltimore: Penguin Books.

Johnson, Lyndon B. 1971. *The Vantage Point*. New York: Holt, Rinehart and Winston.

Marmor, Theodore R. 1970. *The Politics of Medicare*. Chicago: Aldine.

Mills, Wilbur. 1964. *Congressional Record*, October 3, pp. 24015–16.

Redman, Eric. 1973. *The Dance of Legislation*. New York: Simon and Schuster.

Starr, Paul. 1982. *The Social Transformation of American Medicine*. New York: Basic Books.

Sundquist, James L. 1968. *Politics and Policy: The Eisenhower, Kennedy and Johnson Years.* Washington: Brookings Institution.

Thompson, Frank J. 1981. *Health Policy and the Bureaucracy: Politics and Implementation.* Cambridge: MIT Press.

Wolkstein, Irwin. 1970. Medicare 1971: Changing Attitudes and Changing Legislation. *Law and Contemporary Problems* 35:697–715.

2

Medicare: The Record to Date

David Blumenthal

Assessing Medicare's contribution to the health and well-being of Americans is no simple task. Available data on the length and quality of life among elderly Americans is insufficient to fully evaluate the effects of this fundamental health care reform. Even where major changes have been documented in the elderly's utilization of health care or in their health status, it is often difficult to say with precision whether or to what extent Medicare was responsible. During the last twenty-three years, many other factors have affected the lives of the aged and their families, including the creation of other governmental programs, such as Medicaid, the rising income of the elderly, the advent of new medical technologies, changes in the diet and smoking patterns of older adults, and changes in the structure of the nuclear family.

Nevertheless, existing information provides some basis for concluding that Medicare has enjoyed a number of successes. These can be grouped into four categories: administrative accomplishments, protection of elders against the cost of illness, improvements in access to health care services, and contributions to the health status of elderly Americans.

The Successes of Medicare

Administrative Acccomplishments

The preoccupation of federal officials with getting Medicare off to a smooth start had at least one salutary effect. The massive administrative problems that might have occurred in the initiation of such an unprecedented federal health program never materialized. By the end of the first year of the program, Medicare had enrolled 19 million elderly American in Part A of the program and a further 17.7 million (93 percent of eligibles) in Part B (Marmor, 1970). Nineteen percent of the enrollees had used Medicare's hospital benefits and 68 percent its physician benefits (Marmor, 1970). In addition to enroling all these individuals and developing systems to pay millions of claims, Medicare had to establish and administer standards certifying the eligibility of participating institutions to receive reimbursement from the program. Given the monumental nature of these tasks, it is not surprising that Medicare delegated some of them to private insurance companies (processing claims) or to state governments (to certify the quality of care in nursing homes). Whatever problems this reliance on private and public agents created, the Social Security Administration's success in getting the program operating quickly must surely rank among the major administrative accomplishments in the recent history of the federal government.

In certain respects, Medicare's administrative record has continued to be impressive. The program has accommodated a 59-percent increase in the number of aged enrollees (who totaled 28.2 million by 1986) as well as the addition of two new categories of beneficiaries: patients with end-stage renal disease, numbering nearly 100,000 by 1986, and citizens with chronic disabilities, numbering nearly 3 million by 1986 (U.S. Department of Health and Human Services, 1985a). In its ability to process claims, Medicare compares favorably with the best private insurance companies, spending an average of 2.5 percent of program costs on administration compared with 7 percent for private companies. Between 1970 and 1984, Medicare's administrative expenditures per claim under Part A dropped from $6.34 to $2.33 in constant 1970 dollars, a fall of 63 percent. Under Part B, costs per claim fell from $3.16 to $0.85 over the same period, a reduction of 84 percent in constant dollars (U.S. General Accounting Office, 1986). Though some observers now feel that Medicare invests too little in program management and that services to beneficiaries may be jeopardized as a result, the federal government and its private contractors can hardly be criticized for managerial profligacy.

Financial Protection for the Elderly

A second accomplishment of the Medicare program has been to protect large numbers of elderly Americans against significant health care expenditures. Whatever gaps persist in such financial protection, there is no question that the elderly would be much worse off today if Medicare did not exist. In 1966, the elderly paid 53 percent of their health care expenditures out-of-pocket compared to 25 percent in 1984 (Table 2–1). For persons 65 and over, Medicare paid for nearly 49 percent of all health care expenditures in 1984, including 75 percent of hospital expenditures and nearly 60 percent of physician care (Table 2–2).

TABLE 2–1 Percentage Distribution of per Capita Personal Health Care Expenditures for Persons 65 Years of Age or Over by Source of Funds, Fiscal Year 1966 and Calendar Year 1984

	1966		*1984*	
Source of Funds	*Amount*	*Percent*	*Amount*	*Percent*
Per capita	$445	100.0	$4,202	100.0
Out-of-pocket	237	53.2	1,059	25.2
Private insurance	71	15.9	304	7.2
Other private	5	1.1	16	0.4
Medicare	—	—	2,051	48.8
Medicaid	—	—	536	12.8
Other government	133	29.8	236	5.6

Source: Adapted from Gornick et al., 1985, p. 52.

TABLE 2–2 Percentage Distribution of per Capita Personal Health Care Expenditures for Persons 65 Years of Age or Over by Source of Funds and Type of Service, 1984

Source of Funds	*Total Care*	*Hospital*	*Physician*	*Nursing Home*	*Other Care*
Amount:					
Per capita	$4,202	$1,900	$868	$880	$554
Percentage Distribution:					
Total	100.0%	100.0%	100.0%	100.0%	100.0%
Out-of-pocket	25.2	3.1	26.1	50.1	59.9
Private insurance	7.2	7.9	13.5	1.1	4.9
Other private	0.4	0.4	0.0	0.7	0.5
Medicare	48.8	74.8	57.8	2.1	19.9
Medicaid	12.8	4.8	1.9	41.5	11.4
Other government	5.6	9.1	0.7	4.4	3.4

Source: Adapted from Gorlick et al., 1985, p. 52.

Improved Access to Health Care

Medicare's third major accomplishment flows from its second. Because of the coverage it has provided, elderly Americans have greater access to health care services than before the program was created. This benefit is most apparent in measures of so-called realized access to care, that is, statistics concerning actual utilization of services (Aday et al., 1980). Between 1967 and 1983, the proportion of elderly Americans receiving hospital services each year increased by 31 percent, from 185 per 1,000 to 242 per 1,000 (Gornick et al., 1985). Because hospitalization rates increased for all demographic groups among the elderly, this change cannot be attributed solely to the aging of the Medicare population. Over this same 16-year period, the number of hospitalizations per 1,000 elderly increased by 42 percent, from 268 per 1,000 to 381 per thousand. Between 1965 and 1975, the rates for cataract operations doubled among the elderly, whereas rates for arthroplasty tripled (Drake, 1978). Despite this increase in access to hospital services, the number of hospital days used each year by the average beneficiary has remained virtually unchanged since the program's enactment, largely because the length of a typical hospital stay has fallen progressively from a peak of 13.8 days in 1967 to 9.1 days in 1984 (Gutterman and Dobson, 1986). Recent reforms in Medicare's methods of paying hospitals have accelerated this fall in length of stay.

The enactment of Medicare has also been associated with increased access to physician services. In 1963, 68 percent of aged, noninstitutionalized Americans saw a physician at least once a year. By 1970, the rate had risen to 76 percent; by 1980, to 82 percent (Gornick et al., 1985). Though the proportion of elderly seeing physicians has increased under Medicare, the average number of visits per aged individual per year has remained unchanged: 6.8 in 1963; 6.7 in 1980.

Similar trends are apparent in use of home health services. Between 1967 and 1983, the proportion of elderly Americans using home health agency benefits under Medicare increased by 608 percent, from 7 to 46 individuals per 1,000 enrollees.

One of the most impressive effects of Medicare (in combination with Medicaid, which covers about 3 million elderly poor) has been to improve access to care among the poor and minority elderly. From 1967 to 1983, the proportion of nonwhite elderly entering a hospital each year increased by 59 percent compared to 30 percent among whites. In 1967, whites were nearly 49 percent more likely than nonwhites to see a physician at least once during each year. By 1983, that disparity had fallen to 10 percent. (Gornick et al., 1985). Fuchs (1986) has noted that after Medicare's enactment, differences in use of surgical services among elders of low and high income narrowed dramatically. Between 1969 and 1976, differences in the rate of use of physician visits among elders with incomes less than $5,000 and those with incomes three to five times greater fell from 26 percent to nearly zero (Link et al., 1982).

Improved Health Status

Some observers feel that increases in utilization of services by elderly individuals are very much a mixed blessing. A substantial portion of those added hospital stays or physician visits may be unnecessary, thus adding to the costs of the program without conferring commensurate health benefits (Califano, 1986; Fuchs, 1986). Though this contention may have some merit, it is also clear that the enactment of Medicare has been temporally associated with considerable improvement in the health status of elderly Americans.

Since 1900, life expectancy at age 65 has increased from 11.9 to 16.8 years (Gornick et al., 1985). Of that gain, 44 percent has occurred since Medicare became law. Between 1965 and 1984, life expectancy at age 65 increased by 15.1 percent in the United States or about 0.79 percent per year. During the 15 years from 1950 to 1965, life expectancy among the elderly increased by only 5 percent or 0.33 percent per year, less than half the rate observed after Medicare's enactment. Since 1968, increases in life expectancy for Americans 65 and older have exceeded those observed among the elderly in most other Western countries (Davis and Rowland, 1986).

There has been some concern that as older Americans live longer they will experience greater disability, that more and more will be living with diseases that formerly would have killed them. Though limited, available data offer some cause for hope on this score. Between 1976 and 1981, the proportion of noninstitutionalized elderly Americans rating their health as fair or poor actually declined somewhat (from 31.3 to 30.1 percent). During that same period, the proportion of noninstitutionalized elderly reporting on national surveys that they were limited by their health in performing a daily activity increased only slightly, from 45.4 to 45.7 percent (U.S. Department of Health and Human Services, 1985b). Rice and Feldman (1983) note that the number of bed-disability days experienced among the average aged American remained unchanged from 1970 to 1980.

Interestingly, the acceleration in the decline in mortality since the mid-1960s has been most striking among the so-called old, old, those over 85 years of age (Rosenwaike et al., 1980). In fact, improvements in death rates for this age group exceeded those for every other age group in the population. According to figures from the National Center for Health Statistics, death rates among Americans over 85 declined by 28.2 percent from 1966 to 1977 compared to only 12.1 percent from 1933 to 1966.

As is true for younger age groups, a large portion of the fall in death rates among the very old can be explained by reduced deaths from heart and cerebrovascular disease (Rosenwaike et al., 1980). In younger age groups, the drop in deaths from heart disease and stroke is attributed in large measure to nonmedical factors, such as changes in diet, physical activity and smoking habits. It is not clear, however, that these modifications in behavior played a comparable role in the improved health of the very old. It remains to be proven, for example, that elderly reaching the age of 85 during the 1970s significantly modified their diets or levels of physical activity during the preceding decade or that, if they did, such behavioral changes would improve longevity in this unique population group. Interestingly, data on smoking patterns among the elderly during this period provide mixed evidence on whether declines in tobacco consumption could explain some of the improvement in the health status of the very old. Among institutionalized American men over the age of 65, the proportion smoking fell from 28.5 to 23.0 percent between 1965 and 1976—and changed hardly at all between 1976 and 1983. But among women in the same demographic group, the proportion of smokers *rose* from 9.8 to 12.8 percent between 1965 and 1976—peaking at 16.8 by 1980 and then declining to 13.1 by 1983 (U.S. Department of Health and Human Services, 1985b). Better access to health care services and better treatment (including treatment of hypertension) seem just as plausible as changes in lifestyle as explanations for the dramatic reduction in cardiovasular death rates among Americans over 85 in the first decade after Medicare's enactment.

The Other Side of the Ledger

Despite these impressive accomplishments, the Medicare program also faces impressive problems, some of which, as noted, can be traced to its original design. Discussed in greater detail in subsequent chapters, these problems can be grouped into four broad categories: problems of excessive cost, inadequate coverage, excessive complexity and unfair treatment of particular groups of elderly or providers.

Excessive Costs

The increasing costs of the Medicare program have received by far the greatest attention from policymakers. From 1967 to 1984, Medicare expenditures increased from $4.7 billion to $64.6 billion, a compounded annual growth rate of 16.7 percent before inflation, or 9.1 percent after inflation is taken into account. Because of this rapid growth rate, Medicare has accounted for an increasing proportion of national health expenditures: 15 pecent in 1967 compared to 26.7 percent in 1984. During this same period, expenditures under Part A grew from $3.4 billion to $43.3 billion and under Part B from $1.2 billion to $19.7 billion, resulting in real compound annual growth rates of 8.6 and 10.3 percent, respectively (Table 2–3).

Some insight into the root causes of these increases in expenditures can be gleaned from examining the contribution of inflation and certain other factors. In a study of hospital costs between 1973 and 1983, the Health Care Financing Administration (HCFA) concluded that general inflation explained 50.9 percent of increases in expenditures, hospital input prices in excess of inflation accounted for 14.6 percent, growth in the number of elderly 6.7 percent, increases in admissions per capita 4.4 percent and increases in "intensity per admission" 23.4 percent (Gornick et al., 1985). Here, intensity is generally taken to mean the number and complexity of services provided during a given hospital admission. A very similar picture emerges from an examination of increases in physician expenditures (see Chapter 6).

TABLE 2-3 Medicare Benefit Payments and Annual Percentage Change, 1966–84

Year	*Total (billions)*	*Hospital Insurance (billions)*	*Supplementary Medical Insurance (billions)*	*Annual Change for Total*
1966	$ 1.0	$ 0.9	$ 0.1	— %
1967	4.6	3.4	1.2	346.5
1968	5.7	4.2	1.5	25.2
1969	6.6	4.7	1.9	15.9
1970	7.1	5.1	2.0	7.5
1971	7.9	5.8	2.1	10.8
1972	8.6	6.3	2.3	9.9
1973	9.6	7.1	2.5	10.9
1974	12.4	9.1	3.3	29.6
1975	15.6	11.3	4.3	25.5
1976	18.4	13.3	5.1	18.2
1977	21.8	15.7	6.0	18.2
1978	24.9	17.7	7.3	14.5
1979	29.3	20.6	8.7	17.6
1980	35.7	25.1	10.6	21.7
1981	43.5	30.3	13.1	21.7
1982	51.1	35.6	15.5	17.6
1983	57.4	39.3	18.1	12.4
1984	62.9	43.3	19.7	9.5
Percent:				
ACRG[a]	16.6	16.1	17.9	—
ACRRG[b]	9.1	8.6	10.3	—

[a]Annual compound rate of growth 1967–84.

[b]Annual compound real rate of growth 1967–84, adjusted for changes in Consumer Price Index 1967–84.

Source: Gornick, et al., 1985, p. 43.

This breakdown into the components of increases in Medicare spending indicates the very important role that systemic inflation, both inside and outside the medical care sector, has played in raising Medicare expenditures. Medicare, it should always be remembered, is part of a much larger health care system and of a still larger economy. The program's problems can never be definitively resolved by actions or policies that affect only Medicare itself.

But the important role of increases in intensity of treatment in raising Medicare expenditures also hints at ways in which Medicare policies themselves contributed to real growth in program expenditures and in general health care spending. There is a general consensus among students of Medicare that until recently the methods by which it paid providers encouraged an unnecessary and unjustified increase in the intensity of treatment provided beneficiaries (see Chapters 5 and 6). By paying hospitals on the basis of retrospectively calculated costs (prior to the enactment of Medicare's Prospective Payment System [PPS] in 1983) and paying physicians on the basis of usual and customary fees, Medicare provided no incentive for providers to take costs into account in deciding whether a given treatment was necessary or appropriate. This problem was compounded by the explosion of new medical technologies, whose use is generously compensated but whose value is often poorly documented or overstated at the time of introduction (Banta et al., 1981; Evans, 1985). It is widely suspected that the improvements in health status associated with Medicare might have been achieved at considerably less cost if the program (and the health care system generally) had paid providers differently.

Increases in Medicare's costs are sometimes attributed as well to the fact that it has insulated the elderly from the financial consequences of using health care services and encouraged them to seek unnecessary services. Providing such financial protection, of course, was an intended consequence of the program, perhaps its most important goal. Nevertheless, it is reasonable to ask whether the program went too far in this direction. However, an examination of the cost burden borne by elderly Americans leaves the impression that, if anything, the opposite is the case. In many ways, the coverage provided by Medicare is still inadequate.

Inadequate Coverage

Twenty-three years after Medicare's enactment, elderly Americans are still exposed to substantial out-of-pocket health care expenditures. If premiums for Part B of Medicare and for supplementary private insurance are included, the elderly in 1984 spent 15 percent of their income on average for health care: about the same as they did in 1966 (Table 2–4). Because health care expenditures (and thus expenditures for insurance as well as for hospital and physician coinsurance and deductibles) continue to rise faster than the income of the elderly, by 1987 the elderly paid more as a proportion of their income for health care services than they did before Medicare's enactment. The Congressional Budget Office estimated in 1986 that the 17 percent of elderly Americans who are hospitalized just once each year would face average out-of-pocket liabilities of $1,360 in 1987 (Gordon, 1986). The deductible payment for a single hospitalization in 1987 was $520. In 1984, elderly Medicare beneficiaries spent an average of $359 out-of-pocket in coinsurance and deductible payments for services nominally covered by Medicare, excluding out-of-pocket payments for such uncovered services as prescription drugs, most long-term care and mental health care (Waldo and Lazenby, 1984).

For a substantial number of elders, a portion of these costs will be covered by their supplementary private plans, or Medigap policies. However, 20 percent of elders have no coverage other than Medicare (Gordon, 1986). What is more, even

TABLE 2–4 Mean Out-of-Pocket Health Costs as a Percentage of Income for Persons 65 Years of Age or Over, Selected Years 1966–84

Year	*Mean Out-of-Pocket Expenditures*	*Mean Personal Income*	*Out-of-Pocket as a Percentage of Income*
1966	$ 300	$ 2,000	15%
1977	690	5,592	12
1981	1,187	8,639	14
1984	1,575	10,615	15

Source: Adapted from Gornick, et al., 1985, p. 53.

Original Source: U.S. Congress, Senate, Special Committee on Aging, 1984.

Medigap policies provide little or no protection against expenditures for long-term care, including long-term nursing home costs and home health care costs. Elderly Americans still pay more than 50 percent of their nursing home expenditures out-of-pocket, and Medicare itself pays only 2.1 percent of those costs. To be eligible for Medicaid coverage of nursing home services, nonpoor elders must first impoverish themselves, a humiliating requirement.

The failure to pay for nursing home care is symptomatic of a more general inadequacy in the Medicare program. Medicare's coverage provisions and cost-sharing requirements were borrowed from private insurance policies available in 1965. At the time, it was generally assumed that elders' health care needs and use were like those of younger Americans. We have learned better since then. Older patients are more likely to have chronic illnesses, multiple conditions, and a complicated interaction of health, social and economic needs. By not adapting to these differences, Medicare has inadvertently left beneficiaries exposed to unacceptably large copayments and left them without coverage for needed services. These problems are greatest for the oldest beneficiaries: one in four elders over the age of 85 requires nursing home care for which Medicare will not pay; the average 85-year-old spends a third of his or her income on health care costs Medicare does not cover. As the average Medicare beneficiary gets older over the next several decades, such inadequacies will become increasingly apparent.

Equally telling, despite the availability of Medigap policies for those who can afford them and Medicaid assistance for the very poor, large numbers of elderly Americans still incur catastrophic health care expenditures each year for acute care services. According to Congressional Budget Office projections, in 1987 nearly 26 percent of the elderly with Medigap policies, about 4.6 million individuals, paid more than $1,000 out-of-pocket for acute health care services (Gordon, 1986).

Program Complexity

The many gaps in Medicare coverage also contribute to a complexity that makes the program unnecessarily difficult to use on a day-to-day basis. There are no simple rules governing Medicare coverage or payment policies. Hospital and physician services are treated quite differently in terms of copayment requirements. For hospital services, the amount patients must pay varies with the number of days in the hospital. Physicians may decide on a visit-by-visit, service-by-service basis whether to accept what Medicare pays as compensation in full or to bill the patient more. Some home health care visits are covered, others are not, depending on complex regulations. Even young and energetic individuals have trouble sorting through their parents' bills when called on to help. The confusion created among isolated elders with impaired eyesight or hearing can be almost overwhelming.

This confusion is further exacerbated by Medicare's administrative structure and by recent cutbacks in the resources available for program management. As already noted, the Medicare program consists in reality of two insurance programs, one for hospital care and one for everything else the program covers. The administration of Part A is delegated to private agents called intermediaries, whereas the administration of Part B is delegated to similar agents called carriers. Though a single company (generally an insurance company) may serve as both carrier and intermediary in a given community, different organizations frequently perform these roles. Thus a given patient with questions or complaints about coverage for a single hospital stay may have to approach two different organizations for information or relief.

The appeals processes to resolve disputes between patients and these private agents also differ for Part A and Part B. Under Part A, appeals involving large sums must be resolved by impartial administrative law judges employed by the federal government. Under Part B, however, appeals are usually considered by hearing officers designated by the carriers, who are often parties to the complaint. To make things even more confusing, patients who feel that they are being forced to leave the hospital too early as a result of Medicare's new PPS must appeal to still a third private entity, newly created Peer Review Organizations (PROs), which now have statutory authority for monitoring the quality of hospital care under the PPS.

In a thorough 1986 study of the administration of Part B of Medicare, the U.S. General Accounting Office (GAO), the investigative arm of Congress, recently reported that the performance of carriers was beginning to decline, perhaps as a result of cuts in funds for administrative support. Between 1980 and 1985, the GAO noted, the average processing time for beneficiary claims increased by 13.8 percent, from 14.3 to 16.6 days. The average processing time for provider claims went up 19.4 percent, from 11.8 to 14.1 days. And the number of claims pending at the end of the year nearly tripled, from 4.4 million to 11 million. If this continues or worsens, these delays can impose financial hardship on beneficiaries awaiting compensation from Medicare for bills they have already paid out-of-pocket. Administrative delays and confusion could also make Medicare patients less attractive to providers over the long term and impair elders' access to care.

Inequities

In addition to these problems of cost, lack of coverage, and administrative complexity, Medicare has failed to ameliorate important inequities among classes of beneficiaries. Though access to care has improved for poor and minority elderly, they continue to use less health care than more-wealthy white citizens over 65. In 1977, the average black Medicare beneficiary visited a physician five times a year compared to more than six times a year for whites (Davis and Rowland, 1986). Income also continues to influence use of services. Adjusting for health status, elderly with incomes below the poverty level use 34 percent fewer physician visits each year than those with incomes more than twice the poverty line.

One reason for this persistent differential in use of services may be that poor and minority elderly are less likely to have the resources to purchase Medigap policies. Premiums for such plans ranged from $100 to $1,000 in 1984 and averaged between $300 to $400 per person ($600 to $800 for an elderly couple). Though Medicaid covers out-of-pocket expenditures for some poor elderly, many do not qualify for such coverage because of very stringent income requirements in some states. As a result, among noninstitutionalized elderly in 1984, nearly 30 percent with incomes below $8,999 dollars lacked either Medicaid or supplementary private insurance, compared to 10 percent with incomes of $25,000 and over (Table 2–5). Interestingly, more vulnerable elderly, those over 80 years of age, were also more likely than the less vulnerable, those 65 to 69 years old, to lack such coverage (26.5 percent vs. 17.3 percent).

TABLE 2-5 Characteristics of Elderly Medicare Enrollees, April 1984[a b]

Characteristic	*Number of Enrollees (millions)*	*Percentage of Enrollees*	*Percentage Having Neither Private Supplementary Coverage nor Medicaid Eligibility*
Total	25.6	100.0%	20.1%
		Family Income	
Under $5,000	3.1	12.2	28.5
$ 5,000– 8,999	5.6	21.8	29.9
$ 9,000–14,999	6.2	24.1	20.8
$15,000–24,999	5.9	22.9	13.7
$25,000 and over	4.9	19.1	10.1
		Age	
65–69	8.6	33.3	17.3
70–74	7.2	28.0	19.1
75–79	4.9	19.3	20.1
80 and above	5.0	19.4	26.5
		Self-Reported Health Status	
Excellent	6.6	25.6	19.5
Good	9.5	37.1	20.1
Fair	6.4	25.2	20.4
Poor	3.1	12.1	20.8

[a]Details may not add to totals because of rounding.

[b]These estimates apply to the civilian, noninstitutionalized population age 65 and over enrolled in Medicare.

Source: Adapted from U.S. Congressional Budget Office calculations based on the Survey of Income and Program Participation and the 1980 National Medical Care Utilization and Expenditure Survey.

Even though they use fewer services, poor elderly are considerably more burdened by out-of-pocket health care expenditures than the nonpoor. In 1980, according to HCFA statistics, 12 percent of poor and near-poor elderly paid more than 15 percent of their income for health care compared with 1 percent of middle-income elderly and 0 percent of those with high incomes (see Chapter 4 for greater detail).

Finally, as later discussion will document, Medicare's methods of paying providers creates inequities in their compensation as well. Once implemented, uniform national rates for paying hospitals (adjusted for diagnosis-related-groups [DRGs]) will result in a substantial bonus for generally less-costly hospitals in the South and West compared to those in the North and East. Similarly, specialists, surgeons and urban physicians have historically received higher payments for comparable services than have primary care practitioners and physicians in rural areas (see Chapters 5 and 6).

With their roots in the history, politics and management of the Medicare program, these problems in its current performance constitute a significant indictment that some detractors have used to justify dismantling the program and the substitution of private alternatives. Although not minimizing the extent of Medicare's failings or the difficulties of positive change, we feel that a balanced view of its accomplishments and shortfalls argue for less drastic measures that will, nonetheless, require creativity and persistence to accomplish.

REFERENCES

Aday, Lu Ann, Ronald Anderson and Gretchen V. Fleming. 1980. *Health Care in the U.S.: Equitable for Whom?* Beverly Hills, CA: Sage.

Banta, H. D., C. J. Behney and J. S. Wilhems. 1981. *Toward Rational Technology in Medicine*. New York: Springer.

Califano, Joseph A. 1986. *The American Health Care Revolution: Who Lives? Who Dies? Who Pays?* New York: Random House.

Davis, K., and D. Rowland. 1986. *Medicare Policy: New Directions for Health and Long-Term Care*. Baltimore: Johns Hopkins University Press.

Drake, D. F. 1978. Does Money Spent on Health Care Really Improve U.S. Health Status? *Hospitals* 52:63–65.

Evans, Robert G. 1985. Illusions of Necessity: Evading Responsibility for Choice in Health Care. *Journal of Health Politics, Policy and Law* 10 (3):439–67.

Fuchs, V. R. 1986. *The Health Economy*. Cambridge: Harvard University Press.

Gordon, N. M. 1986. Testimony before the Subcommittee on Health and the Environment, Committee on Energy and Commerce. U.S. Congress, House of Representatives, March 26.

Gornick, Marian, Jay N. Greenberg, Paul W. Eggers et al. 1985. Twenty Years of Medicare and Medicaid: Covered Populations, Use of Benefits, and Program Expenditures. *Health Care Financing Review, 1985 Anuual Supplement*, pp. 13–59.

Guterman, S., and A. Dobson. 1986. Impact of the Medicare Prospective Payment System for Hospitals. *Health Care Financing Review* 7 (3):97–114.

Link, C. R., S. H. Long and R. F. Settle. 1982. Equity and Utilization of Health Care Services by the Medicare Elderly. *Journal of Human Resources* 17 (2):195–212.

Marmor, Theodore R. 1970. *The Politics of Medicare*. Chicago: Aldine.

Rice, D. P., and J. J. Feldman. 1983. Living Longer in the United States: Demographic Changes and Health Needs of the Elderly. *Milbank Memorial Fund Quarterly* 61 (3):362–96.

Rosenwaike, I., N. Yaffe and P. C. Sagi. 1980. The Recent Decline in Mortality of the Extreme Aged: An Analysis of Statistical Data. *American Journal of Public Health* 70 (10):1074–80.

U.S. Department of Health and Human Services. Health Care Financing Administration, Bureau of Data Management and Strategy. 1985a. *HCFA Statistics*. HCFA Pub. No. 03209.

———. 1985b. National Center for Health Statistics, Public Health Service, DHHS. Pub. No. (PHS) 86–1232 *Health United States, 1985*.

U.S. General Accounting Office. 1986. *Medicare. Existing Contract Authority Can Provide for Effective Program Administration*.

Waldo, D. R., and H. C. Lazenby. 1984. Demographic Characteristics and Health Care Use and Expenditures by the Aged in the United States: 1977–1984. *Health Care Financing Review* 6 (1):1–29.

3

Beneficiary Cost Sharing in the Medicare Program

MARK SCHLESINGER
PAMELA BROWN DRUMHELLER

Medicare was created to provide the elderly with the financial protection of health insurance. For a variety of reasons, including both conscious design and political compromise, beneficiaries were asked to pay a portion of their health care costs out of their own pockets in the form of premiums and copayments.

Medicare's cost-sharing arrangements were intended to work in conjunction with Medicaid, which was passed as companion legislation. A cooperative program between state and federal government, Medicaid provides additional coverage for the poor and for those with very large health care expenses. This combined arrangement between Medicare and Medicaid was designed to meet three goals.

Goals of Medicare's Cost-Sharing Arrangements

Financial Protection

As is true of all insurance policies, the principal goal of Medicare's cost-sharing design was to provide beneficiaries with protection against severe financial loss. Prior to Medicare's passage, few elderly persons could obtain affordable private health insurance. As a result, over a third of all elders who were hospitalized in 1962 spent at least 25 percent of their income on medical care (Kovar, 1986). In the words of Senator Edward Kennedy (1986, p. 11), then newly elected to Congress, "In the dark days before Medicare, senior citizens lived in fear that a single illness could wipe out a lifetime of savings and transform the dream of a comfortable retirement into a nightmare of poverty and despair."

To address this concern Medicare applied the broadest and most generous coverage to hospital care, the source of the largest medical bills. Nonetheless, Congress recognized that because Medicare does not cover all health care costs, beneficiaries could still be liable for financially devastating health care bills. Thus a provision was included in the Medicaid program that allowed state legislatures to provide additional financial protection by permitting Medicare beneficiaries to spend down to Medicaid eligibility; that is, to deduct medical bills from their income in determining whether they meet income-based eligibility requirements for Medicaid. In states with spend-down provisions, elders with large medical bills can thus, in principle, become eligible for Medicaid benefits even if they are not poor.

Control of Program Costs

A second goal of Medicare's design was to encourage beneficiaries to use only needed services. If insurance covered all of the costs of health care, beneficiaries would have no financial incentive to conserve on their use of health services and, indeed, might use services that have costs far greater than the benefits they offer. Thus Medicare, like almost all private insurance, requires that enrollees pay for some of the costs of the care they receive through deductibles and coinsurance.[1] Within each benefit period of Medicare's Part A coverage, which primarily covers hospital care, beneficiaries must pay a deductible roughly equal to the average cost of 1 day in the hospital.[2] For the first 60 days of coverage in a benefit period, there is no coinsurance. Coverage between the 60th and 90th days has a 25 percent coinsurance rate; coverage beyond 90 days has a 50 percent coinsurance. Under Part B, which primarily covers physician services, beneficiaries face a $75 annual deductible and 20 percent coinsurance for each service delivered once coverage begins.

Fair Share of Costs for Beneficiaries

Unlike private insurance, Medicare's cost-sharing arrangements were also shaped by what were seen as basic principles of fairness, particularly a concern that out-of-pocket expenses for health care be affordable to all elders. Private insurance premium rates are set to cover the cost of the health care that enrollees use, less coinsurance and deductibles. However, because many elders incur substantial health care expenses, it was generally agreed that if Medicare premiums were set to cover the full cost of Part B services, they would be beyond the financial means of many elders. To avoid this, Congress chose to have elders pay only one-half the costs of Part B coverage through premiums, subsidizing the rest through general federal revenues. Part A is financed through payroll taxes and has no premium.

Over the past few decades, Congress has twice changed the way in which Part B premium rates are set in an attempt to ensure that elders continue to pay a "fair share" of program costs. "Fair" in this context has had two quite different meanings. On one hand, "fair" meant a share that did not exceed the financial resources of the elderly as a group. Concerned that health care costs were rising far faster than elders' incomes, Congress amended the Social Security Act in 1972 to limit the annual growth of Part B premiums to the cost-of-living increases in Social Security payments. As a result, premiums as a portion of Part B costs fell from 50 percent in 1966 to 25 percent in the mid-1980s. This decline evoked concern over "fair share" in a second sense: that elders pay an adequate share of the overall costs of the program so that younger generations are not asked to pay too much for the health care of their parents. In 1986, Congress changed the criteria for annual charges in Part B premiums and required that they be raised to maintain a 25-percent contribution.

The costs borne by beneficiaries have thus reflected changing congressional perceptions of how best to determine an equitable contribution from elders. Cost sharing provisions have also reflected other aspects of this concern for equity, particularly the need to ensure that all elders had reasonable access to medical providers. For example, Congress gave doctors the option to bill patients for more than the amount that Medicare would reimburse (that is, to not "accept assignment" of charges) (Thompson, 1981). It did so in part because it was feared that physicians would be unwilling to treat beneficiaries for the fees Medicare would pay. Beneficiaries whose doctors do not accept assignment thus must pay physician charges for their medical care in addition to Medicare's coinsurance and deductibles (see Chapter 6). Though initially small, by 1983 these unassigned charges had grown to be as large in aggregate as beneficiaries' liability for coinsurance on Medicare-covered physician's services (Waldo and Lazenby, 1984).

Partly as the result of such unexpected increases in costs, elders' expenses from using health services have become far larger than had been anticipated in 1965. Some observers charge that under these circumstances cost-sharing provisions that initially appeared sensible are now unfair, ineffective or counterproductive. These concerns are described in detail in the following section. In the subsequent section, we will review reforms that have been proposed to address these perceived shortcomings. The chapter concludes with a discussion of some broader perspectives on reform of Medicare's cost-sharing arrangements.

References will be found throughout this chapter to "the burden of Medicare cost sharing" on the elderly. This phrase refers to the total costs paid by beneficiaries for health care services covered by Medicare, including Part B premiums, unassigned physician charges and deductibles and coinsurance for both Parts A and B. Most assessments of Medicare's cost-sharing provisions treat Parts A and B separately, rarely view copayments as a contribution to Medicare program costs (as they do not appear in the federal budget) and often omit entirely the role of unassigned charges. Although Medicare's Parts A and B have different cost-sharing requirements, we believe that it is important to assess the consequences of all cost-sharing, both to accurately calculate the burden borne by beneficiaries, and to fairly assess their contribution to the costs of services covered by Medicare.

Shortcomings of Medicare's Cost-Sharing Provisions

Rapid Increases in Program Spending

Medicare program costs have increased from $4.5 billion in 1967 to $72 billion in 1985 (Waldo et al., 1986). Much of this dramatic growth is due to the inflation of medical prices that has beset all purchasers of health care (Arnett et al., 1985). But Medicare's cost increases have not resulted solely from higher medical prices, as evidenced by the fact that Medicare costs are growing faster than those of privately insured younger populations. Over the past 15 years, hospital expenditures for the elderly have grown 50 percent faster than for those under 65, even taking into account the rising average age of beneficiaries (U.S. Department of Health and Human Services, 1984). Physician spending has grown even faster.

How did this happen? Were Medicare's copayments too small to induce beneficiaries to be prudent purchasers? Were they misconceived or misapplied? The answer is a complicated one.

By almost any standard, deductibles and coinsurance charges have been large enough to discourage beneficiaries from unnecessary use of health care. Medicare's copayment rates are high compared to those of private insurance. Even though private insurers have recently increased copayments to hold down costs, the cost sharing required of working Americans is still less stringent than that faced by their retired parents. Medicare's hospital deductible in 1986 was $492, rising to $520 in 1987. In contrast, the latest national survey of private insurance plans shows that the average deductible was less than $150 a year (Glenn and Brazda, 1985c). Only about 10 percent of all private insurance plans had copayment rates as high as 20 percent, yet Medicare beneficiaries pay 20 percent of every physician bill.

Medicare's copayments are also large enough to affect beneficiaries' use of health care. Copayments have limited the elderly's use of physicians' services more than that of hospital care, but they have constrained the use of each (Link et al., 1982; Wan, 1982). Surveys indicate that the elderly are more sensitive to the cost of hospital care than any other age group (Inguanzo and Harju, 1985).

Increases in Medicare spending, then, are not due to inadequate copayments but rather to two other sources. First, the majority of elderly beneficiaries do not pay Medicare's coinsurance and deductibles. Excluding those elders who are enrolled in the Medicaid program, more than two thirds of all Medicare beneficiaries purchase private supplementary insurance, sometimes called Medigap plans (Health Insurance Association of America, 1983; Gordon, 1986). These plans pay almost exclusively for Medicare deductibles and coinsurance (Cafferata, 1984; Rice and Gabel, 1986). Not surprisingly, the elderly who have Medigap coverage are more likely to use health services. Comparing equally healthy elders, those with Medigap plans received 25 percent more hospital and physician care than those covered by Medicare alone (Long et al., 1982).

The number of beneficiaries who purchase supplementary insurance continues to increase over time. Between 1969 and 1981, for example, the proportion of beneficiaries with Medigap coverage of nonsurgical physician charges grew from 13 to 41 percent (U.S. Department of Health, Education and Welfare, 1973; Health Insurance Association of America, 1983). Increased purchase of these plans can thus account for some of the rapid increase in program spending.

Beneficiaries' use of health care is also a result of decisions made by providers, decisions that seem to play a more important role in driving up Medicare's costs than do choices made by consumers. Medicare spending on physician services is the fastest growing area of program costs. After adjusting for inflation, these costs have grown 9 percent a year between 1975 and 1985 (U.S. Congressional Budget Office, 1986). The average beneficiary, though, visited a physician no more often in 1985 than in 1975. Virtually all the increase in inflation-adjusted spending came from growth in the number of tests and procedures ordered by physicians during each visit (U.S. Congress, Senate, Special Committee on Aging, 1984). Even the most prudent consumer of health care services has little control over these costs.

To summarize, Medicare has relied primarily on copayments to control program spending. This strategy proved inadequate, in part because beneficiaries avoided this cost sharing by purchasing private insurance and in part because much health care spending is controlled by providers rather than by patients. Ways of compensating for increased program costs owing to purchase of Medigap policies are discussed later in this chapter. Strategies for creating more effective incentives for providers to control costs are addressed in Chapters 5, 6 and 7.

Inadequate Financial Protection

As an insurance program, Medicare should provide beneficiaries adequate protection against the financial risks of health care costs. These costs present two threats to patients' financial security. Because health services can be very expensive, particularly for those most seriously ill, they can exceed the savings of even the most prudent families. In addition, because illness is unpredictable, health costs can be difficult to budget, especially for individuals with limited incomes.

Medicare does not provide sufficient protection against either of these financial threats. Because the bulk of beneficiaries' costs for services covered by Medicare are incurred when they use services, these expenses are as unpredictable as illness itself. Unassigned physician charges are perhaps the most unpredictable form of cost sharing facing beneficiaries. Physicians can ask elders to pay these charges for any given bill; statistics show that beneficiaries are as likely to face unassigned charges for very large bills as for small ones (Burney and Schieber, 1985). Several years ago, the Health Care Financing Administration (HCFA) began a voluntary program in which participating physicians agreed to accept assignment in return for favorable administrative treatment. Though assignment rates went up as a result, freezes on Medicare's reimbursement for physicians over the past two years have angered many physicians, and participation rates in the voluntary assignment program fell as much as fourfold in some states in 1986 (Riffer, 1986).

Beneficiaries' share of health care costs can all too easily become a catastrophic financial burden. Because beneficiaries face open-ended liability for medical bills—in fact, the hospital coinsurance rate goes up the longer the beneficiary is hospitalized—Medicare provides very limited protection against the costs of very serious or chronic illness. Five percent of all beneficiaries, about 1.5 million elders a year, are hospitalized twice a year, and those who do not have Medigap insurance incur on average over $3,000 in out-of-pocket expenses under Medicare's cost-sharing provisions (Rice and Gabel, 1986).[3] Half a million beneficiaries pay over $2,000 out-of-pocket a year in Medicare copayments alone, exclusive of unassigned charges and premiums (U.S. Congressional Budget Office, 1983). This is almost a quarter of the income of the average elder (U.S. Congress, House, Select Committee on Aging, 1985).

The problem of catastrophic costs has been exacerbated by the failure of Medicaid to provide reliable protection for the medically needy. This failure occurred because the medically needy program was left as an option for individual states and, faced by rapidly rising Medicaid costs, only 30 states chose to participate (Sawyer et al., 1983).[4] In addition, the generosity of the existing programs varies tremendously. About half set the income level at which beneficiaries become medically needy below what the state considers "poor" for other programs and purposes (Davidson and Marmor, 1980). In these states, families have to be literally destitute before qualifying as medically needy.

The current threats to elders' financial security can be reduced in three ways: by setting a limit on total copayment liability in a given year, reducing copayments overall, or requiring that Medicaid provide a uniformly more generous medically needy program. The merits of each approach are discussed later in this chapter.

Inequitable Distribution of Program Costs

As noted earlier, past congressional actions suggest that legislators believe that a "fair" sharing of costs requires both that beneficiaries make an adequate contribution to program spending and that these costs do not exceed their financial resources. Over the past two decades, one of these goals has been achieved, the other has not.

The program has been quite successful in maintaining beneficiaries' contribution to the costs of Medicare. Including premiums, copayments and unassigned charges, beneficiaries have annually paid between 25 and 30 percent of the combined costs of Part A and Part B over the past two decades.

Initially, the program was also able to ensure that health care costs did not become excessively burdensome to the elderly. During Medicare's first decade, beneficiaries' spending on health care (including long-term care) as a fraction of their income actually declined, from 15 percent in 1965 to 12 percent in the mid-1970s. Since that time, however, health care expenses have risen faster than elders' incomes. As a result, by the mid-1980s, the portion of beneficiaries' incomes spent on health care costs was the same as before the enactment of the Medicare program. According to current projections, the aggregate burden of health care spending will be considerably larger by 1990 (Table 3-1).

This increased burden occurs largely because much of beneficiaries' cost sharing is paid through copayments that are set as a fraction of health care charges. These grow as quickly as medical care prices and much faster than elders' incomes. The portion of beneficiaries' costs paid through copayments has been rapidly increasing over time. In 1968, copayments accounted for one-half beneficiaries' spending on cost sharing. By 1983, the portion spent on copayments had increased to two thirds of cost sharing spending (Waldo and Lazenby, 1984).

TABLE 3–1 Changes Over Time in the Fraction of Medicare Beneficiaries' Income Spent on Health Care Costs

Year	*Percentage of Mean Income*
1965	15.0%
1977	12.3
1984	14.6
1990	18.9

Source: Adapted from U.S. Congress, House, Select Committee on Aging. 1985.

TABLE 3–2 Per Capita Health Care Costs for Noninstitutionalized Elders by Income Level (1984 dollars)

Income Class[a] (*% of population*)	*Out-of-Pocket Expenditures* (*% of income*)	*Part B Premiums*[b] (*% of income*)	*Medigap Premiums*[c] (*% of income*)	*Total Health Care Costs*[d] (*% of income*)
Poor/Near-poor (26 percent)	$807 (16.7%)	$136 (3.1%)	$329 (6.8%)	$1272 (26.6%)
Low-income (24 percent)	$819 (5.1%)	$164 (1.1%)	$433 (2.7%)	$1416 (8.9%)
Moderate-income (30 percent)	$777 (2.8%)	$168 (0.7%)	$600 (2.3%)	$1416 (5.8%)
High-income (20 percent)	$896 (1.4%)	$171 (0.4%)	$642 (1.1%)	$1709 (2.9%)

[a]Poor/near-poor elders have incomes less than 125 percent of the poverty line; low-income elders, between 125 and 200 percent; moderate-income elders between 200 and 300 percent; high-income elders have incomes greater than 300 percent of poverty line.

[b]Part B prekiums were $172.80 annually for all enrollees. The difference in average expenditures across income classes reflects the extent to which Medicaid covers the costs of these premiums.

[c]Cafferata reports average premiums for a combined category of poor/near poor/low income. For these calculations, it is assumed that poor and low income have the same average premiums; the differences in average expenditure reflect differences in the extent to which elders purchase Medigap policies.

[d]Reported values for out-of-pocket and Medigap spending are based on findings of the 1977 National Medical Care Expenditure Survey increased to 1984 levels and based on data reported by Waldo and Lazenby. Percentage of income adjusted in based on aggregate changes reported by U.S. Congress, House, Select Committee on Aging, 1985.

Sources: U.S. Congress, Senate, Special Committee on Aging, 1984; McMillan et al., 1983, p. 9; Cafferata, 1984, p. 9).

This growing cost burden is most problematic for those least able to pay for health care. Medicare treats all beneficiaries alike, charging them the same premiums and copayments. Not all, however, have equal financial resources. About a quarter of all beneficiaries have incomes less than 125 percent of the poverty line. On average, these elders spend over a fourth of their income annually on health care and health insurance (Table 3-2). If the costs of nursing home care are included, the proportion is as high as 40 percent of income (ICF, 1985). These poor elderly spend ten times as much of their income on medical care as do elders with incomes in the highest quartile.

Financial pressures are greatest on the oldest beneficiaries, who have the fewest financial resources and incur the greatest health care costs. Elders over the age of 85 are four times as likely to live in poverty as those age 65 (ICF, 1985) and spend more than twice as many days in the hospital each year (Soldo and Manton, 1985). As a result, beneficiaries 85 and older spend almost 40 percent of their income on health care and health insurance (Table 3-3).[5] The proportion of Medicare beneficiaries over 85 has doubled since the program was enacted; it will double again within the next quarter century (Rosenwaike, 1985). Medicare's failure to adequately protect this group will thus become of increasing public concern.

These inequities have developed in part because Medicaid has not provided adequate financial protection for low-income elders. Concerned with rising Medicaid costs, states have contained spending by restricting eligibility. In the 1970s, a decade of high inflation, states could limit their Medicaid expenditures simply by failing to increase their eligibility standards (the highest income at which individuals

TABLE 3–3 Out-of-Pocket Expenses as a Fraction of Beneficiaries' Income by Age of Beneficiary, 1986

	Health Care Spending	
Age Range	*Excluding Private Insurance Premiums*	*Including Private Insurance Premiums*
65–69	4.2%	6.5%
65+	8.6	11.6
85+	37.5	41.7

Source: ICF, 1985.

could qualify for coverage) to keep pace with the rising cost of living (Granneman and Pauly, 1983). As a result, the proportion of the low-income population covered by Medicaid fell sharply between the mid-1970s and 1980s (Munnell, 1985b). By the early 1980s, less than 40 percent of the elderly population with incomes below the poverty line were covered by Medicaid (McMillan and Gornick, 1984).

To correct these inequities, the Medicaid program could be reformed so that it more adequately covers low-income beneficiaries. Alternatively, Medicare's cost-sharing provisions could be adjusted to take beneficiaries' financial resources into account. The advantages and disadvantages of each of these approaches will be discussed later in this chapter.

An Emerging Complexity

Though long debated, the final legislation that created Medicare was hastily assembled. As a result, the two parts of the program have different structures, financing sources, regulations and cost-sharing provisions. For example, Part B coverage was borrowed from the Federal Employees' Health Benefits Plan, whereas the entire Medicaid program was a last-minute addition, modeled on prior federal initiatives.

This made cost-sharing requirements complicated from the beginning. The program incorporated four different types of copayments. Hospital deductibles and coinsurance were based on the somewhat confusing concept of a benefit period, defined as a length of time after an initial hospitalization. Unassigned charges could be imposed at physicians' discretion. In addition to these provisions, beneficiaries are asked to understand Medicaid eligibility requirements and the often complex exclusions and provisions of private supplementary policies.

The problems resulting from complicated cost sharing requirements are increasing over time. Unassigned charges have grown from a relatively trivial expense to a cost as large as Medicare's formal Part B coinsurance. A growing number of elders purchase several Medigap plans, often with overlapping coverages. All too often, these multiple policies are simply too complicated for beneficiaries to understand (Firman, 1985; McCall et al., 1986). Because it is so difficult to determine what their cost-sharing liabilities are under Medicare or how these interact with other coverages, beneficiaries may fail to use needed health care or may not be reimbursed for treatment they do receive (Feder and Holahan, 1979).

Thus, although program simplicity was not an explicit goal of Medicare's designers,[6] it is increasingly seen as a valid objective for reform. A number of the proposals intended to meet other goals also simplify cost-sharing provisions. Others may make cost sharing more complicated and confusing. In assessing these proposals, we will consider their effects on both beneficiaries' understanding of the program and the costs that beneficiaries are likely to face.

Options for the Reform of Medicare's Cost-Sharing Provisions

In response to shortcomings in Medicare's cost-sharing arrangements, proposals have been developed to better control program costs while offering Medicare's beneficiaries greater financial security within a more equitable, simpler program. A number of specific reforms have been proposed toward each of these ends.

Adjust Cost Sharing to Control Spending

Increase Beneficiaries' Premiums and Copayments

In the face of growing program costs, it has been proposed that Medicare raise premiums or copayments. Higher premiums could be used to reduce the burden of Medicare spending on taxpayers. Higher copayments would encourage beneficiaries to further limit their use of health care services. As previously noted, though, beneficiaries' health care costs are already higher in relation to income than before Medicare was enacted. Whether cost sharing should be increased still further is a matter of considerable debate.

Those who favor increased cost sharing claim that the elderly are now receiving more and better health care than when Medicare was initiated. "We should keep in mind the tremendous range and intensity of services made available by the program to the elderly today compared to eighteen years ago" (Dole, 1984, p. 3). Certainly, Medicare has enhanced beneficiaries' access to health care. However, use of health care by the elderly has remained relatively stable over the past decade. The number of physician visits and the length of hospital stays have not increased since the mid-1970s. Between 1972 and 1982, the average number of physician visits per year by Medicare beneficiaries declined from 5.0 to 4.6 (U.S. Congress, Senate, Special Committee on Aging, 1984). The average number of days in the hospital for those over the age of 65 declined from 3.0 to 2.9 between 1977 and 1982 (U.S. Department of Health and Human Services, 1984).

It is true that once beneficiaries are in a physician's office or admitted to a hospital, they may, indeed, receive a higher intensity of medical services than they did two decades ago. However, this higher intensity is, for the most part, a result of the fact that physicians perform more tests and procedures than they did twenty years ago. Increasing copayments is not likely to affect these costs and forces the elderly to pay for physician practices over which they have little control.

A second justification offered for increasing beneficiaries' share of program costs is that the financial burden imposed by Medicare cost-sharing requirements has been overestimated by calculations that include services not covered by Medicare, such as nursing home care (Dole, 1984). Indeed, if one eliminates the costs of nursing home care from beneficiaries' out-of-pocket expenditures (see column 2 in

Table 3–4), the overall burden on beneficiaries declines and the apparent performance of Medicare over the past twenty-three years improves.

Nonetheless, even excluding nursing home expenses, the portion of income that beneficiaries will spend on health care by 1990 (13.2%) will exceed the portion of income spent before Medicare was enacted (12.2%). Moreover, the costs of nursing home care place a very real financial burden on America's elders that should not be ignored.

Finally, it has been argued that because the overall financial situation of the elderly has improved since 1965, beneficiaries can afford to pay more of their income for health care. "In America today, there are those who claim that the elderly are 'well-off' and can easily afford to absorb cutbacks in Social Security, Medicare and Medicaid" (Roybal, 1986, p. 2). Far fewer elders have incomes below the poverty line today than in 1965. In the early 1960s, roughly one third of all elders were classified as "poor," twice the rate of younger Americans. Two decades later, the poverty rate among the elderly had fallen to less than 15 percent, about equal to that of other age groups (Aiken and Bays, 1984).

Although the number of elderly persons living in poverty has declined, many still have very low incomes. Roughly half of all elders and almost 60 percent of those over the age of 75 have incomes below twice the poverty line (Atkins, 1985). The limited financial resources of the average Medicare beneficiary can be appreciated by considering the burden of health care costs on an elderly person with a median income, a statistic that is not distorted by the small number of elders with extremely large incomes.[7] As Table 3–4 demonstrates, this burden has grown rapidly over the past decade; a beneficiary with a median income in 1984 paid more than 20% of his or her income for health care.

It may be helpful to view this burden in slightly different terms by considering the typical budget of a Medicare beneficiary with a median income. Table 3–5 has been constructed using data collected by the Department of Labor. An elderly person in 1980–81 had a median income of about $7,100 after taxes. The annual costs of the bare necessities (food, shelter and transportation) were over $6,100 (U.S.

TABLE 3–4 Changes Over Time in the Fraction of Medicare Beneficiaries' Income Spent on Health Care Costs

	Measured in Terms of Beneficiaries'		
Year	*Mean Income Spent on Health Care*	*Mean Income Spent on Health Care with no Nursing Home Costs*	*Median Income Spent on Health Care*
1965	15.0%	12.2%	— %
1977	12.3	7.9	18.5
1984	14.6	9.9	21.4
1990	18.9	13.2	27.7[a]

[a]Data published in the Select, Committee on Aging (1985) report did not include projection for median income to 1990. The projection presented here assumes that the distribution of income for the elderly remains the same in 1990 as in 1984.

Sources: Costs as a fraction of mean and median income from U.S. Congress, House, Select Committee on Aging, 1985. Costs without nursing home expenses calculated by using data from ICF, 1985.

TABLE 3–5 Health Care Spending and the Average Elder's Discretionary Income, 1980–81

Type of Spending	*Amount Spent by Average Elder in $5,000–$10,000 Income Bracket*[a]	
Average after-tax income		$7,143
Total spending for necessities		6,137
Food	2,116	
Shelter and utilities	2,606	
Transportation	1,415	
Discretionary income		1,006
Health care and health insurance		949

[a]Published spending figures available only by income bracket. the elder with median income in 30 percent of all elders fell within this bracket.

Source: U.S. Department of Labor, 1985.

Department of Labor, 1985). This does not include the costs of clothing or other necessary expenditures. This left roughly $1,000 a year in discretionary income. In 1980–81, the average elderly person with a median income spent $949 on health care. Hence, increasing Medicare cost sharing is likely to force many beneficiaries to spend less on necessities like food and shelter.

It has also been proposed that Medicare add new copayment charges or raise existing ones to further discourage the use of unnecessary medical care and thereby reduce program costs. In its 1984 budget proposal, for example, the Reagan administration recommended adding coinsurance to the first 60 days of hospital coverage. Added cost sharing, proponents argued, would motivate patients who are not seriously ill to keep their hospital stays short (Brazda and Glenn, 1983). A similar recommendation was made in the same year by the Advisory Council on Social Security Reform. Congress recently approved a Reagan administration proposal to increase the Part B deductible and index it so that it grows at the same rate as health care costs increase.

Increasing copayments would almost certainly reduce elders' use of health care. Large copayments, however, may discourage needed treatment as much or more than unnecessary use of health services.[8] Medicare's hospital deductible in 1987 was almost $520; as a result, an elder hospitalized just once in a year will incur $1,500 in expenses owing to cost sharing and uncovered services (Gordon, 1986). Table 3–5 suggests that any further copayment charges will make copayments so large relative to the average elder's discretionary income that they will constitute a significant financial barrier to using health care for many beneficiaries.

Additional copayment charges are most likely to affect beneficiaries with low incomes who cannot afford to purchase Medigap insurance. Beneficiaries who have Medigap policies often pay no copayments at all (Cafferata, 1984) and use significantly more health services (Link et al., 1982). Younger and wealthier beneficiaries purchase Medigap policies more frequently than do other elders (Long et al., 1982); elders with annual incomes of $25,000 are twice as likely to purchase supplementary insurance as are those with incomes of $5,000 a year (Gordon, 1986).

The poorest elderly, therefore, bear the brunt of Medicare's copayments, yet these beneficiaries are already less likely to receive needed health care than are their better-off counterparts (Branch and Nemeth, 1985). Increasing copayments will only add to this disparity.

Increase Cost Sharing for Purchasers of Medigap Policies

Supplementary insurance policies increase Medicare program costs by paying beneficiaries' copayments and thus removing the incentive to limit unnecessary use of health care services. Increasing cost sharing for beneficiaries who purchase Medigap policies would be a more equitable and effective way of controlling program costs than raising Medicare copayments for all the elderly. Two approaches have been proposed. The first would impose a tax on the actuarial value, or premiums, of Medigap policies equal to the additional costs that they create for the Medicare program (Long and Smeeding, 1984; Munnell, 1985a). Such a tax would increase the price of Medigap insurance policies by about 30 percent (Ginsburg, 1983). The tax revenues could be used to offset the costs to the Medicare program (see Chapter 8).

As a source of revenue, such a tax would be fairly progressive. Because elders with higher incomes purchase more comprehensive policies, the costs of this tax are distributed somewhat more equitably in relation to income than is a flat premium for all beneficiaries (Long and Smeeding, 1984). Nonetheless, elders in the lowest income quintile who hold Medigap policies would pay, as a fraction of income, seven times as much in taxes as would those in the upper quintile (Long and Smeeding, 1984). As a result, it is the poorest beneficiaries who would be most likely to give up their Medigap policies.

A second approach is to prohibit private insurers from offering first-dollar coverage or to limit coverage to a small number of prototype policies that leave some copayments uncovered. This strategy would be a more direct, effective and equitable means of preserving Medicare's copayment incentives than taxes that increase the costs of Medigap policies.

Such a regulatory approach might, however, face challenges. Insurance has traditionally been regulated by the states, and federal limitations on insurance coverage could be contested as an infringement on state authority. This problem could be avoided by following the model of the 1982 Baucus amendments to the Social Security Act that made certain federal funding contingent on state regulation of Medigap policies. In so doing, regulatory authority was left at the state level. The drawback, however, is that state compliance is ultimately voluntary and may be adopted by states only sporadically. As an alternative, it has been proposed that the federal government offer a public supplementary policy through the Medicare program. This option will be discussed later in this chapter.

Increase Beneficiaries' Financial Security

As noted earlier, beneficiaries' financial security can be enhanced both by limiting the probability that they will face catastrophically large expenses and by making moderate expenditures more predictable. The first two proposals discussed here limit beneficiaries' financially catastrophic expenditures, whereas the third proposal would make out-of-pocket expenses more predictable.

Establish Ceilings on Copayment Liability

The cost-sharing reform most often recommended for the Medicare program is the creation of a ceiling, or cap, on copayment liability (Ball, 1984; Hsiao and Kelly, 1984; Davis and Rowland, 1986). Such an arrangement would, in effect, extend insurance coverage to protect beneficiaries against accumulating large medical bills for services covered by Medicare.[9] Beneficiaries would pay copayment charges until their total spending on copayments for the year reached a specified dollar amount. Once the ceiling was reached, copayment charges would be paid directly by the Medicare program. This additional coverage would be financed wholly or partly through monthly premiums paid by beneficiaries.

The desire for financial protection is so great among the elderly—and so intrinsic to the principles of insurance on which Medicare is formulated—that a ceiling on copayments is certain to generate bipartisan political support (U.S. Congress, House, Select Committee on Aging, 1985).[10] A simple cap on liability for all beneficiaries would not create great administrative burdens; the U.S. Congressional Budget Office (CBO) (1983, p. xviii) reports that "it would be easy to limit the amount of Medicare-related costs required of any beneficiary in a year."

However, two controversial questions concerning a cap on copayment liability must be resolved. The first is whether catastrophic coverage should be made a mandatory part of the Medicare program or offered as voluntary policy either through the Medicare program or through private insurers. The second issue concerns the dollar amount at which a ceiling on liability should be set.

Proponents of a voluntary approach argue that purchase of coverage should not be required of beneficiaries. Catastrophic coverage would add a new Medicare premium of between $80 and $150 a year—depending on the level at which liability was capped—to enrollees' out-of-pocket costs. Not all elders may be willing or able to spend this much. If coverage is voluntary, elders can decide for themselves whether the coverage is worth the cost. If private insurers provide catastrophic coverage, elders will be able to select among several plans and choose the policy that best meets their needs and financial resources.

The liability of any voluntary approach is that catastrophic coverage is most likely to be purchased by elders who will have above-average health care expenses. As a result, premium rates may be considerably higher than if costs were spread among all Medicare beneficiaries. Coverage provided through private insurers would add even more to the cost of catastrophic protection. The administrative and marketing costs of private insurance are significantly higher than the administrative costs of the Medicare program (Blair and Vogel, 1975). As a result, private plans marketed to individual beneficiaries would carry premiums $30 to $60 higher than those Medicare would require for the same coverage. These considerations strongly argue for a mandatory federal program.

The principal debate over including a catastrophic ceiling in the Medicare program involves setting the level of the cap. Some proposals would limit copayment liability to as little as $500 a year, whereas others allow as much as $2,500. The lower the ceiling, the more extensive the financial protection but the more costly the reform. A cap would increase program expenses both because Medicare would pay some of the costs previously borne by the elderly as copayments and because once beneficiaries exceeded the ceiling, they would have no financial incentive to limit their use of additional health services. The U.S. Congressional Budget Office (CBO) (1983) has predicted that capping copayment liability at $1,000 a year would cost the program $4 to $5 billion annually and that setting the cap at $2,000 would reduce costs by about half.

Capping copayments thus creates a dilemma. If the ceiling is set too high, it provides inadequate financial protection. If the ceiling is set too low, it may result in unnecessary use of health care and certainly will lead to large increases in the costs of the Medicare program.

There are two ways around this dilemma. The first would adjust the copayment ceiling to beneficiaries' income (Hsiao and Kelly, 1984). This would provide financial protection for beneficiaries at a lower cost to the program than a uniform cap as the cap could be set higher for beneficiaries with substantial incomes (U.S. Congressional Budget Office, 1983). An income-adjusted cap would, however, be more difficult to administer (Davis and Rowland, 1986). The problems of income-based adjustments to cost sharing are discussed in greater detail later.

A second strategy for creating a more equitable copayment ceiling is to establish separate caps for hospital and ambulatory care.[11] Because hospital treatment is so expensive, many elders would reach the limits of a combined ceiling in a single admission. Separate caps would provide protection against the high costs of inpatient care while maintaining a financial incentive for prudent use of outpatient services. Because hospital care is less likely to be at the discretion of the beneficiary than a visit to a physician's office, the hospital cap could be set at a relatively low level without encouraging a great deal of unnecessary use of health care services.

The principal liability of setting separate caps is that it will add to the complexity of the program. A confusingly complex reform will do little to increase beneficiaries' sense of financial security (Hagen, 1986).

Require Greater Uniformity in Medicaid Eligibility

Medicare and Medicaid were intended to jointly provide a coherent, equitable pattern of cost sharing. Owing to political and fiscal pressures to limit Medicaid program costs, however, Medicaid became the weak link in this scheme.

Significant interstate variation has developed within the Medicaid program. In states with the most generous eligibility (Rhode Island, California and Hawaii), Medicaid covers more than 75 percent of the state's residents with incomes below the poverty line. In contrast, in the least generous states (Texas, Wyoming, Idaho and South Dakota), 20 percent or less of the poor population are eligible for Medicaid (U.S. Department of Health and Human Services, 1985). Some states do not offer a medically needy program, and others impose very strict limitations on eligibility for medically needy status. In 1984, the state with the most stringent medically needy program required that a family of two spend all but $1,600 in annual income on health care before becoming eligible for Medicaid. This was less than a quarter of the income protected by the most generous state, which set eligibility at an annual income of $6,936 for a family of two (U.S. Department of Health and Human Services, 1985). Thus, beneficiaries in some states face far greater risks to financial security than do those in other states with more generous programs.

To provide greater financial protection and to reduce inequities, a number of proposals have been formulated to increase the uniformity of Medicaid eligibility.

Some call for a federal requirement that all states meet more generous nationwide standards for eligibility (Davis and Rowland, 1986). Others suggest that the federal government assume responsibility for a portion—either acute or long-term care coverage—of the Medicaid program (National Study Group on State Medicaid Strategies, 1983).

Proposals requiring greater uniformity and generosity in the Medicaid program are likely to meet resistance for two reasons. First, over the past few years, the trend in the administration of the Medicaid program has been toward allowing greater variability at the state level (Granneman and Pauly, 1983; Glenn and Brazda, 1985b). In 1981, Congress gave states the option of setting different levels of eligibility for different groups that might qualify under their medically needy program. Over the past several years, states have been allowed to waive various requirements that had previously been imposed on all state programs. This shift in policy has coincided with reduced rates of growth in Medicaid costs and "many state officials credit the new cost containment to waivers and other measures allowing greater program flexibility" (Glenn and Brazda, 1985b, p. 1). It may, therefore, be difficult to develop political support for any proposal that reverses this trend by imposing uniform federal eligibility requirements.[12]

Second, such requirements would certainly increase the budgets of both the federal and state governments as well as reduce states' fiscal flexibility. If Medicaid eligibility were, for example, set nationwide at 125 percent of the poverty line for elders, states' Medicaid expenditures would increase by $2 billion to $3 billion a year for acute care services alone (Harvard Medicare Project, 1986). Further, restricting eligibility has been the principal means by which states have been able to control their Medicaid costs when economic downturns limit their tax revenues (Munnell, 1985b). Whether or not such restrictions are appropriate or acceptable, states are likely to resist proposals that limit their ability to control Medicaid costs (Davidson et al., 1986).

It is possible, however, that this resistance could be reduced if long-term care spending were no longer a responsibility of Medicaid. States are currently facing rapidly increasing long-term care costs under the Medicaid program as the American baby-boom population ages (Vladeck and Firman, 1983). The costs of acute care coverage are more stable and also predictable than are costs for long-term care, which tend to be more dependent on the availability of formal and informal services for impaired elders (Doty, 1986). Eliminating responsibility for long-term care would present a major saving to the states, and these additional revenues could well be used to finance increases in eligibility for Medicaid coverage of acute care services.

Reduce or Eliminate Unassigned Physician Charges

Reducing or eliminating unassigned physician charges would increase financial security for beneficiaries and reduce inappropriate constraints on the use of health services. Options for achieving this are discussed in greater detail in Chapter 6. We focus here briefly on the implications of these reforms for beneficiaries.

Regardless of the specific approach used, requiring physicians to accept Medicare's fees as payment in full would reduce beneficiaries' access to health care by causing some doctors to refuse to treat the elderly (Mitchell and Cromwell, 1983). The extent of this problem, however, could be reduced in several ways. First, assignment could be required only for specialists and surgeons. It is these physicians whose bills impose the largest burden on the elderly (Burney and Schieber, 1985). Limiting mandatory assignment to these doctors would also avoid disrupting elders' relationship with their primary care providers.

Second, delaying the implementation of this reform will reduce the probability that physicians will refuse to treat Medicare enrollees. The number of physicians continues to increase and will do so in the future. Past studies have found that the more physicians there are in the community, the less likely they are to refuse to treat Medicare enrollees if required to accept assignment (Paringer, 1980; Mitchell and Cromwell, 1983).

Even with these ameliorative strategies, there may be some regions of the country in which access to care would be jeopardized if physicians refused to participate in a Medicare program with mandatory assignment. This is most likely to occur in rural areas or low-income communities where there are relatively few physicians within easy travel of the elderly. It may thus make sense to treat these physicians differently, much as Medicare's hospital payment system now gives special treatment to institutions that are the sole providers of care in their community (see Chapter 5).

Adjust Cost Sharing to Promote a Fair Share of Beneficiaries' Costs

When the Medicare program was first enacted, Congress considered a proposal to vary copayments with the income of the beneficiary (Marmor, 1970). Sponsored by Senator Abraham Ribicoff, this proposal gained considerable political support and was only narrowly defeated. It lost because the Kennedy administration favored a program that treated all elders identically in hopes of gaining broader political support for Medicare. Income adjustments were also viewed by many as unnecessary as the elderly were at the time being portrayed politically as a group that was almost uniformly needy (Binstock, 1985).

As the economic well-being of the elderly has improved over the past two decades, however, policymakers in Washington have become increasingly aware of differences in financial resources among Medicare enrollees. As a result, particularly in the past four years, Congress has become more receptive to proposals that would adjust Medicare cost sharing according to beneficiaries' incomes (Glenn and Brazda, 1985a). These proposals fall into three categories: those that adjust copayments to income, those that adjust premiums to incomes (either directly or indirectly through the tax system), and those that would establish a means test for Medicare eligibility.

In general, these proposals have met with three types of criticism: (1) income adjustment will increase the costs and complexity of program administration, (2) income adjustment may stigmatize those beneficiaries it is intended to help by identifying them as having low incomes, and (3) such reforms could undermine Medicare's long-term political stability by reducing the extent to which wealthier and more politically active Americans support the program. These criticisms are more applicable to some forms of income adjustment than to others.

Adjust Copayments to Income

If copayments are to encourage prudent use of health services without inhibiting access to care, they should reflect differences in beneficiaries' responsiveness to financial incentives. As one would expect, individuals with low incomes decrease their use of health services to a greater extent when faced with copayments than do those with higher incomes (Lohr et al., 1986). Consequently, if the appropriate incentives for use of health care are to be maintained, copayment charges should increase with an enrollee's income.

Calculating this adjustment for elders who file tax returns would not be difficult. However, fewer than half of all Americans over the age of 65 are required to file tax returns. Determining the income of the remainder would add to the administrative costs of the Medicare program, perhaps by as much as 50 percent (Conrad and Marmor, 1983).

The billing process would be more complicated and costly than the present system because copayment charges for a given service would differ for beneficiaries in different income brackets. In addition, because billing for copayments for Part B services is done by physicians (who accept assignment) rather than by Medicare, physicians would have to be informed of the correct copayment rate for each patient. This is not only administratively cumbersome for physicians, but also means that physicians would be privy to information about their patients' incomes.

A third difficulty is that many believe that income is not an adequate measure of financial resources and that the value of elder's financial assets and property should be considered when determining their cost-sharing liability. This leads to a number of problems. Policymakers disagree about the extent to which the value of beneficiaries' homes—the principal asset for most elders—should be included in such a calculation, as this may force some elders to sell their homes (Davidson and Marmor, 1980). Including assets in a measure of elders' financial means also creates an incentive for them to transfer assets to their children, causing an asset test to understate their true financial resources (Wetle, 1985). Finally, obtaining accurate current information on the value of beneficiaries' assets would add to Medicare's administrative burden.

Some of these problems can be avoided if, rather than adjusting copayments for each service delivered, a ceiling on copayments is adjusted to enrollees' incomes. Beneficiaries would pay copayment charges until the cap for their particular income level was reached, at which time copayments would be eliminated. This arrangement saves administrative costs because it does not involve adjusting every bill. Although providers would be notified by Medicare when a beneficiary's copayment ceiling was reached, they would not have explicit information about beneficiaries' incomes. This approach, however, neither avoids the problems of obtaining information about income from elders who do not file tax returns nor ameliorates controversy over how to measure financial resources.

ADJUST PREMIUMS TO INCOME

Premiums can be adjusted to income in several ways. The existing Part B premium (as well as any new premiums) could simply be set as a proportion of each beneficiary's income. Alternatively, premiums could either be replaced or supplemented by income-based taxes that would be earmarked for financing the Medicare program.

Adjusting premiums, as opposed to copayments, has the advantage of not informing providers about beneficiaries' incomes. In addition, because premiums are more predictable than copayments, beneficiaries can more easily assess and budget for their cost-sharing responsibilities. The other strengths and weaknesses of adjusting premiums depend on the specific approach used.

Income-related premiums, like income-related copayments, would add to Medicare's administrative costs because the program would need information about all beneficiaries' incomes. In addition, such a reform could undermine political support for Medicare. Beneficiaries who had higher incomes during their working years contributed more to the program in payroll taxes than did those with lower incomes. Middle and high-income beneficiaries might thus view income-related premiums as an unfair financial burden. Some policymakers believe that if the burden on upper-income elders becomes too great, they may no longer actively support the program, narrowing its political base (Krizay and Wilson, 1974). This would reduce the support of those elders who are likely to be the most politically active and effective.

Several proposals have called for replacing the existing Part B premium with an income-related tax. In 1985, a White House policy group called for eliminating the premium and for taxing the actuarial value of Medicare benefits as a form of income (Glenn and Brazda, 1985a). This would involve calculating the dollar value of annual use of health services covered by Medicare and treating some or all of this value as taxable income. A number of academic studies have considered replacing the Part B premium with a separate income tax surcharge for the elderly that would be earmarked for financing the Medicare program (Davis and Rowland, 1984; Long and Smeeding, 1984).

Tax-based proposals have some generic advantages over the direct adjustment of premiums to beneficiaries' income. Tax-based financing would involve no additional administrative costs for the Medicare program because revenues would be collected by the Internal Revenue Service (IRS). An income tax surcharge would impose minimal burdens of paperwork on the elderly as it would apply only to those with taxable income. Taxing the actuarial value of Medicare benefits would require more elders to file income tax returns because their Medicare benefits would be counted as income, but it would not affect the beneficiaries whose income remained below taxable levels (see Chapter 8 for additional discussion of these proposals).

Taxing the actuarial value of Medicare benefits has some additional political liabilities. First, because medical prices rise far faster than elders' incomes (U.S. Congress. House. Select Committee on Aging, 1985), the actuarial value of Medicare benefits is likely to become an even larger source of tax liability for the elderly. Elders may see this as a significantly greater threat to their financial security than would be a tax surcharge set as a fixed percentage of tax liability. In addition, proposals for taxing the actuarial value of Medicare benefits may be perceived as the first step in taxing the insurance benefits of working-age Americans, which would be opposed by organized labor.

Whatever the approach, completely replacing premiums with taxes could undermine Medicare's political stability. Medicare is a popular program in part because it is seen as a form of health insurance, a product that all Americans clearly need and value. Elders' payment of regular premiums reinforces this image. If premiums are completely eliminated, Medicare might be perceived by taxpayers as simply another program of governmental spending.

This problem could be avoided if taxes supplemented rather than replaced existing premiums. Several bills have been introduced in Congress that would supplement the Part B premium with a special tax set as a proportion of beneficiaries' income. A mixed system of cost sharing, in which beneficiaries contributed in part through a flat premium and in part through earmarked income taxes, could increase the equity of cost sharing without significantly affecting the overall image of the program. To partially base elders' contributions on income might increase support among the general public by counteracting the impression that younger taxpayers are inappropriately being asked to subsidize elders who are already financially well-off.

MEANS-TEST MEDICARE ELIGIBILITY

Means-testing Medicare eligibility, that is, allowing only elders with incomes or financial resources below a certain level to participate in the program, has not been widely advocated. However, the idea was broached by the Office of Management and Budget in 1982 and the Congressional Budget Office in 1983. Although it met with strong initial resistance in Congress, legislators seem to be increasingly willing to consider such proposals in recent years (Glenn and Brazda, 1985a).

Means testing would create some administrative costs for the program as HCFA would need to determine elders' incomes to assess eligibility. However, means-testing eligibility would probably not require that more elders file tax returns to report their income. Eligibility limits are likely to be set high enough, so that they would only affect elders who were already filing tax returns.

If Medicare benefits were limited only to low-income elders, though, it would undoubtedly stigmatize those beneficiaries who qualified for the program and might discourage them from enrolling (see Chapter 4). Means testing also creates serious risk for the long-term political stability of the Medicare program. Means testing could alter the popular perception of Medicare in a serious and lasting fashion—from that of a social insurance program to a welfare program. This change would drastically reduce political support for the program. Finally, means testing would raise difficult questions about program financing. It would be difficult to justify continued payroll-tax contributions to a program for which the taxed might not later be eligible.

Simplify Cost-Sharing Responsibilities

ELIMINATE UNNECESSARY COPAYMENTS

Perhaps the most important purpose of copayments is to create incentives for appropriate use of health services. Those that do not foster more appropriate use of care simply add unnecessarily to the complexity of the program. From this perspective, a case can be made for eliminating several of Medicare's existing copayments.

The first is hospital coinsurance. Because coinsurance begins after 60 days of hospitalization, elders who incur this liability are typically very ill. Almost invariably, how and where they are treated is their physician's decision, not their own. Financial incentives have at most a small effect on their use of services.

Hospital coinsurance, moreover, is outdated. In 1965, when these copayments were introduced, hospitals were reimbursed on the basis of costs and providers had no incentive to conserve on hospital spending. Since 1983, however, prospective payment based on diagnostic-related groups (DRGs) has given hospitals a strong financial incentive to limit patients' length of stay (see Chapter 5). Part A coinsurance is therefore unnecessary. Abandoning this form of copayment would simplify the administration of the program and eliminate a major portion of the open-ended liability that beneficiaries now face (Gornick et al., 1983).

It can also be argued that the Part B deductible creates inappropriate incentives for health care use. Because elders tend to disregard symptoms of illness as simply a part of growing old, many do not seek care in a timely fashion (Minaker and Rowe, 1985). Among beneficiaries older than 70 years old, 17 percent fail to seek medical care when they feel ill. These are disproportionately the poorest elders (Branch and Nemeth, 1985). By discouraging beneficiaries with low incomes from seeking treatment, the Part B deductible may delay needed care and make eventual treatment more costly and less efficacious.

The deductible is also inequitable for beneficiaries because it influences the behavior of only some elders. Elders with chronic illnesses or disability—about half the Medicare population—visit a physician between 8 and 10 times a year (Butler and Newacheck, 1981). Because these enrollees know they will use far more than the cost of the deductible each year, the deductible does not create a disincentive for using health care. In contrast, elders without chronic illnesses visit physicians an average of 2 to 3 times a year, almost all of which (given current physicians' fees) must be paid by the beneficiary under the deductible.[13]

Eliminating the Part B deductible would increase health care use and program costs. However, elders would still be required to pay coinsurance on physician care, thus preserving financial incentives to use care prudently. Moreover, because many elders purchase Medigap policies that cover the cost of the deductible, doing away with it would lead to increased use of health care services for less than half of the enrolled population (Cafferata, 1984).

One objection to eliminating these copayments is that even if they do not encourage more efficient use of health care, they provide an important means of paying for Medicare-covered services. It may, therefore, be desirable to increase beneficiaries' premiums to offset reduced copayments.

Even if premiums were increased, so that beneficiaries' aggregate contribution to Medicare spending was the same as before copayments were eliminated, elders would clearly benefit from this shift. Dollar for dollar, premiums present fewer problems for Medicare enrollees than do copayments. Premium costs are known in advance and can be incorporated into an elder's budget for the month. Premium costs are fixed over a given year and so cannot accumulate to catastrophic levels. Finally, as discussed earlier, premiums can be more readily adjusted than can coinsurance and deductibles to take into account elders' financial resources.

Combine Parts A and B of Medicare

Medicare's separate Parts A (mandatory hospital insurance) and B (optional supplementary medical insurance) are the products of compromise, accident and inertia, not considered planning. In large part the separation resulted from the unexpected addition of coverage for physician services to the original Medicare bill, which covered only hospital care and skilled nursing home services. Legislators at the time took for granted that Medicare would be modeled on existing private health insurance. Private plans in 1965 typically offered separate policies with different terms for hospital and physician coverage, a pattern exemplified by the separation, until recently, of the Blue Cross and Blue Shield organizations. Although the original division is understandable, today the split between Parts A and B makes Medicare needlessly complicated in operation and confusing to its beneficiaries, 97 percent of whom elect Part B coverage (Waldo and Lazenby, 1984).

It has been proposed that Parts A and B of the Medicare program be combined (Ball, 1984). In addition to simplifying the structure of the program and making it easier for beneficiaries to understand, this would also facilitate simpler and more rational cost-sharing requirements. A single Medicare premium could be paid by all beneficiaries as a source of financing for the entire program. This premium might also be used to pay for elimination or reductions of Part A copayments.

Offer A Public Supplementary Insurance Policy

Medigap plans add greatly to the complexity of beneficiaries' cost-sharing arrangements. In conjunction with Medicare's own limitations, the fine print of Medigap policies can make it more difficult for beneficiaries to determine for which costs they are liable and which will be paid by Medicare or Medigap (DeNovo and Shearer, 1978; Feder and Holahan, 1979). The policies themselves are confusing, with many detailed exclusions and specifications (Firman, 1985; Hagen, 1986; McCall et al., 1986).

Federal regulations under the Baucus amendments have undoubtedly reduced some of this confusion by requiring that private supplementary plans cover certain minimum benefits. Nonetheless, considerable confusion still persists among beneficiaries (Hagen, 1986), and elders continue to purchase several private policies, often with overlapping coverages (Rice and Gabel, 1986).

Given these circumstnces, it may be desirable to have the federal government offer its own supplementary policy as an extension of Medicare coverage (DeNovo and Shearer, 1978).[14] Such a plan could be designed to reduce many of the copayments now required but preserve small deductibles or low levels of coinsurance to provide financial incentives for prudent purchase of care (Harvard Medicare Project, 1986).

A public substitute for private policies offers a number of advantages. It would lessen confusion for beneficiaries, giving them a simple option for reducing copayments. It could be provided at lower cost because it would avoid many of the marketing expenses associated with private insurance (Blair and Vogel, 1975). It could also, if desired, be provided on a subsidized basis to beneficiaries with lower incomes, reducing some the inequities that are a part of the current system.

A proposal of this sort, though, would face some opposition. It is likely to be opposed vigorously by the insurance industry. This reform would also increase the overall size of the Medicare budget. Even if this increase were financed entirely through premiums, a larger budget may be viewed as undesirable. Finally, this approach conflicts with the current political preference for relying on the private sector to provide services (Savas, 1982). These objections could be mitigated by using private insurers as fiscal intermediaries as in the Medicare program generally.

Broader Perspectives on Cost-Sharing Reform

In the preceeding pages, we have discussed the advantages and disadvantages of a number of specific proposals. In evaluating the potential for reform of Medicare's cost-sharing provisions, however, it is helpful to keep in mind several broader issues.

First, changing conditions have created both the opportunity and the need for cost-sharing reform. Several provisions that were at one point viewed as reasonable compromises among conflicting goals are problematic today. Beneficiaries currently pay unassigned charges because Congress wished to model Medicare on private insurance and was concerned that physicians might otherwise refuse to treat the elderly, thus reducing access to services. Beneficiaries faced open-ended hospital copayments as a check on uncontrollable expenditures under the original cost-based system of hospital payment that gave hospitals a blank check for extended treatments. Because there is now much less chance of physicians' refusing to treat elder patients and because we now pay hospitals prospectively, the rationales for these forms of cost sharing have become weak or have disappeared. After more than 20 years, it is time to take stock and eliminate these outmoded provisions from the Medicare program.

Second, choosing the best strategy of reform often involves deciding whether changes should be made within or outside the Medicare program. Copayment liability could be limited through a Medicare cap, private insurance policies, or an enhanced medically needy program in Medicaid. Ineffective and inequitable copayment arrangements could be addressed either by increasing Medicare's copayments or by taxing or regulating private supplementary insurance.

Whatever the merits of each individual reform, it is clear that strategies set outside the Medicare program have a number of generic strengths and weaknesses. Working outside the program offers greater potential for adapting reforms to the individual situations of elders while preserving Medicare's tradition of equal treatment of beneficiaries. Through the use of the tax system, income-based cost sharing could be introduced with less risk of stigmatizing beneficiaries or disrupting political support for Medicare. Reforms that can be incorporated into the existing administrative systems of either the Medicaid program or the IRS may avoid costly duplication of administrative mechanisms.

There are, however, some disadvantages in going outside the Medicare program. When cost-sharing arrangements are divided among several programs and cut across tax and health care systems, it may become difficult to coordinate or even assess the effects of changes over time. Provisions outside the Medicare program may also be more subject to political manipulation and thus less reliable over the long term. For example, as a result of state budget pressures, the provisions for the medically needy in the Medicaid program never developed sufficiently to provide adequate financial protection against large medical expenses. Similarly, if a part of the beneficiaries' contribution to Medicare were made through earmarked taxes, program revenues might be affected by every new tax reform package considered in Congress.

Finally, though we have considered them individually, a number of reforms could be readily integrated into packages addressing common goals. For example, cost sharing could be shifted from copayments to premiums by eliminating those copayments that seem inappropriate or counterproductive (e.g., hospital coinsurance, Part B deductible) and increasing premiums to cover the added program costs. In so doing, the program could be made better for beneficiaries without additional cost to taxpayers.

Capping copayment liability would also be less expensive if it were linked to proposals eliminating inappropriate copayments. It has been estimated that these changes in copayment provisions would cut the costs of a copayment ceiling by as much as half (Harvard Medicare Project, 1986). In addition, because adjusting premiums to beneficiaries' incomes is more administratively feasible than adjusting copayments, shifting cost sharing from copayments to premiums facilitates reforms that would more equitably distribute costs among beneficiaries.

By taking advantage of these complementary relationships among proposals, the prospects for meaningful reform can be improved by simultaneously adopting a set of changes rather than by considering each desired reform individually. This integrated approach to reform offers the potential for significant improvements in the ways in which beneficiaries share in the costs of the Medicare program.

NOTES

1. A deductible is the amount of money a beneficiary must spend out-of-pocket for health care before insurance coverage goes into effect; coinsurance is the portion of the bill for each covered service that the beneficiary must pay.

2. A benefit period begins with an episode of hospitalization and ends 60 days after a patient is discharged. Thus, if a patient is readmitted within 2 months after leaving the hospital, the deductible does not apply. The deductible is actually calculated by multiplying $45 by the ratio of hospital costs per day in the current year to costs per day in 1966. Because $45 was approximately the charge for an average hospital day in 1966, the deductible today remains at about the average per diem charge for a hospitalized patient.

3. Using a somewhat different method of calculation, ICF, Inc., a Washington consulting firm estimated that a beneficiary with $10,000 in medical expenses in a year would have only 60 percent paid by Medicare (ICF, 1985). Roughly 5 percent of Medicare's beneficiaries incur medical expenses this large in the course of a year (U.S. Congressional Budget Office, 1983).

4. Five states that do not have medically needy programs allow individuals to spend down to the level at which they would have categorical eligibility.

5. Even if the costs of nursing home care are excluded, about a third of the income of this age group is devoted to health care spending.

6. As noted in Chapter 1, the complexity of the program was raised as a concern in the Senate's debate over the legislation. Because those in the Kennedy administration had focused their thinking on Medicare as a relatively simple program that covered only hospital services, they gave this issue relatively little thought.

7. The mean income, presented earlier, tends to be biased upward by the relatively small number of elders with large incomes. The median captures the average elder in the sense that 50 percent of the elderly have incomes below the median and 50 percent above. In 1984, elders' mean annual income was $10,438, their median income $7,131 (U.S. Congress, House, Select Committee on Aging, 1985).

8. Recently published results from the Rand Health Insurance Study found that non-elderly patients who paid copayments have as high a proportion of "inappropriate" hospitalizations as those who faced no hospital copayments (Siu et al., 1986).

9. It has also been argued that capping copayment liability would reduce the need for beneficiaries to purchase supplementary insurance (Hsiao and Kelly, 1984). In our assessment, however, it is unlikely that limiting liability would have much effect on the purchase of Medigap coverage. Few beneficiaries have policies that provide any real protection against catastrophic costs (Cafferata, 1984). Most elderly seem to purchase Medigap policies in search of first-dollar coverage; a cap on liability would not provide such coverage. A cap on copayment liability is thus not likely to reduce greatly the purchase of private policies (Ginzberg, 1984).

10. Copayment ceilings were included in proposals developed in 1986 by Secretary Otis R. Bowen of the Department of Health and Human Services (DHHS) and by the Democratic-controlled Ways and Means Committee of the House of Representatives.

11. Lave (1986) proposed a similar split cap, putting prescription drugs under one cap and all other services under another.

12. Mandating nationwide changes in eligibility is not, however, without recent precedent. In 1984, Congress required that all states provide Medicaid coverage for certain groups of pregnant women with limited incomes.

13. Because the financial incentives of copayments are felt most by elders with limited incomes, studies have found that, for a given level of health status, beneficiaries' utilization increases with income. However, utilization is unrelated to income if they have a chronic illness (Link et al., 1982).

14. A similar, though more restrictive proposal was made in 1983 by the Advisory Council on Social Security Reform. This group recommended that a first-day hospital coinsurance be introduced for those beneficiaries who did not purchase Part B coverage.

REFERENCES

Aiken, L. H., and K. D. Bays. 1984. The Medicare Debate—Round One. *New England Journal of Medicine* 311 (18):1196–1200.

Arnett, R. H., C. S. Cowell, L. M. Davidoff et al. 1985. Health Spending Trends in the 1980's: Adjusting to Financial Incentives. *Health Care Financing Review* 6 (3):1–27.

Atkins, G. L. 1985. The Economic Status of the Oldest Old. *Milbank Memorial Fund Quarterly* 63 (2):395–419.

Ball, R. M. 1984. *Improving Our National Health Insurance Program.* Paper presented to Conference on Health Financing Policies and Politics, Washington, June 11.

Binstock, R. H. 1985. The Oldest Old: A Fresh Perspective or Compassionate Ageism Revisited. *Milbank Memorial Fund Quarterly* 63 (2):420–51.

Blair, R. D., and R. J. Vogel. 1975. *The Cost of Health Insurance Administration.* Lexington, MA: Lexington Books.

Branch, L. G., and K. T. Nemeth. 1985. When Elders Fail to Visit Physicians. *Medical Care* 23 (11):1265–76.

Brazda, J., and K. Glenn. 1983a. Medicare: Sharing the Costly Burden. *Washington Report on Medicine and Health*, February 21.

Burney, I., and G. Schieber. 1985. Medicare Physicians' Services: The Composition of Spending and Assignment Rates. *Health Care Financing Review* 7 (1):81–96.

Butler, L. H., and P. W. Newacheck. 1981. Health and Social Factors Relevant to Long-Term Care Policy. In *Policy Options in Long-Term Care*, ed. J. Meltzer, F. Farrow and H. Richman, pp. 38–77. Chicago: University of Chicago Press.

Cafferata, G. 1984. *Private Health Insurance Coverage of the Medicare Population: Data Preview 18.* U.S. Department of Health and Human Services, Public Health Service, Office of the Assistant Secretary for Health, National Center for Health Services Research.

Conrad, D., and T. R. Marmor. 1983. Patient Cost Sharing. In *Political Analysis and American Medical Care*, ed. T. R. Marmor, pp. 207–36. Cambridge: Cambridge University Press.

Davidson, S. M., and T. R. Marmor. 1980. *The Cost of Living Longer: National Health Insurance and the Elderly.* Lexington, MA: D. C. Heath.

Davidson, S. M., J. Cromwell, and R. Schurman. 1986. Medicaid Myths: Trends in Medicaid Expenditures and the Prospects for Reform. *Journal of Health Politics, Policy and Law* 10 (4):699–728.

Davis, K., and D. Rowland. 1984. Medicare Financing Reform: A New Medicare Premium.

Proceedings of the Conference on the Future of Medicare. Subcommittee on Health, Committee on Ways and Means. U.S. Congress, House of Representatives, 149–161.

———. 1986. *Medicare Policy: New Directions for Health and Long-Term Care*. Baltimore: Johns Hopkins University Press.

DeNovo, A., and G. Shearer. 1978. *Private Health Insurance to Supplement Medicare*. Volume 1, Policy Planning Issues Paper, Federal Trade Commission.

Dole, R. 1984. Keynote Speech presented at the Government Research Corporation's Ninth Annual Leadership Conference, Washington, June 11.

Doty, P. 1986. Family Care of the Elderly: The Role of Public Policy. *Milbank Memorial Fund Quarterly* 64 (1):34–75.

Feder, J., and J. Holahan. 1979. *Financing Health Care for the Elderly: Medicare, Medicaid, and Private Health Insurance*. Washington: Urban Institute Press.

Firman, J. 1985. Health Care Cooperatives: Innovations for Older People. *Health Affairs* 4 (1):50–61.

Ginsburg, P. B. 1983. Market-Oriented Options in Medicare and Medicaid. In *Market Reforms in Health Care: Current Issues, New Directions, Strategic Decisions*, ed. J. A. Meyer, pp. 103–18. Washington: American Enterprise Institute for Public Policy Research.

Ginsberg, E. 1984. Response to Hsiao and Kelley, *Proceedings of the Conference on the Future of Medicare* Subcommittee on Health, Committee on Ways and Means. U.S. Congress, House of Representatives, 49–54.

Glenn, K., and J. Brazda. 1985a. Medicare and Beneficiary Income. *Washington Report on Medicine and Health*, March 25.

———. 1985b. Medicaid Spending Slows Down. *Washington Report on Medicine and Health*, May 20.

———. 1985c. Health Benefits: Employers in the Driver's Seat. *Washington Report on Medicine and Health*, July 8.

Gordon, N. M. 1986. Testimony before the Subcommittee on Health and the Environment, Committee on Energy and Commerce. U.S. Congress, House of Representatives, March 26.

Gornick, M., J. Beebe and R. Prihoda. 1983. Options for Change Under Medicare: Impact of a Cap on Catastrophic Illness Expense. *Health Care Financing Review* 5 (1):33–43.

Granneman, T. W., and M. V. Pauly. 1983. *Controlling Medicaid Costs: Federalism, Competition, and Choice*. Washington: American Enterprise Institute for Public Policy Research.

Hagen, R. 1986. Medigap Insurance: Pitfalls and Progress. *Business and Health* 3 (5):25–30.

Harvard Medicare Project. 1986. *Medicare: Coming of Age. A Proposal for Reform*. Boston: Division of Health Policy Research and Education, Harvard University.

Health Insurance Association of America. 1983. *Source Book of Health Insurance Data: 1982–1983*. Washington: Author.

Hsiao, W. C., and N. L. Kelly. 1984. Restructuring Medicare Benefits. *Proceedings of the Conference on the Future of Medicare*. Subcommitee on Health, Committee on Ways and Means. U.S. Congress, House of Representatives, 30–48.

ICF Incorporated. 1985. *The Role of Medicare in Financing the Health Care of Older Americans*. Paper submitted to the American Association of Retired Persons, July.

Inquanzo, J., and M. Harju. 1985. What Makes Consumers Select a Hospital? *Hospitals* 59 (6):90–94.

Kovar, M. G. 1986. Expenditures for the Medical Care of Elderly People Living in the Community in 1980. *Milbank Memorial Fund Quarterly* 64 (1):100–32.

Kennedy, E. M. 1986. Testimony U.S. Congress, before the Select Committee on Aging. House of Representatives. Hearing, July 30, 1985.

Krizay, J., and A. Wilson. 1974. *The Patient as Consumer*. Lexington, MA: D.C. Heath.

Lave, J. R. 1986. *The Structure of the Medicare Benefit Package Evolution and Options for Change*. Paper prepared for Conference on What We Have Learned from Twenty Years of Medicare: Implications for Public and Private Policy. University of Pennsylvania, October 8–10.

Link. C. R., S. H. Long and R. F. Settle. 1982. Equity and the Utilization of Health Care Services by the Medicare Elderly. *Journal of Human Resources* 17 (2):195–212.

Lohr, K., R. Brook, C. Komberg, et al. 1986. Use of Medical Care in the Rand Health Insurance Experiment. *Medical Care* (Supplement) 24 (9):531–38.

Long, S. H., R. F. Settle, and C. R. Link. 1982. Who Bears the Burden of Medicare Cost Sharing? *Inquiry* 19 (3):222–34.

Long, S. H., and T. M. Smeeding. 1984. Alternative Medicare Financing Sources. *Proceedings of the Conference on the Future of Medicare*. Subcommittee on Health, Committee on Ways and Means. U.S. Congress, House of Representatives, 168–186.

Marmor, T. R. 1970. *The Politics of Medicare*. Chicago: Aldine.

McCall, N., T. Rice and J. Sangl. 1986. Consumer Knowledge of Medicare and Supplemental Health Insurance Benefits. *Health Service Research* 20 (6):633–57.

McGuire, T. G. 1981. *Financing Psychotherapy: Costs, Effects, and Public Policy*. Cambridge, MA: Ballinger.

McMillan, A., and M. Gornick. 1984. *A Study of the Elderly Medicare—Medicaid Crossover Population Living in the Community*. Health Care Financing Administration Draft.

McMillan, A., P. L. Pine, M. Gornick et al. 1983. A Study of the Crossover Population: Aged Persons Entitled to Both Medicare and Medicaid. *Health Care Financing Review* 4 (4):19–37.

Minaker, K. L., and J. W. Rowe. 1985. Health and Disease Among the Oldest Old: A Clinical Perspective. *Milbank Memorial Fund Quarterly* 63 (2):324–349.

Mitchell, Janet B., and Jerry Cromwell. 1983. Impact of an All-or-Nothing Assignment Requirement Under Medicare. *Health Care Financing Review* 4 (4):59–78.

Munnell, A. H. 1985a. Paying for the Medicare Program. *New England Economic Review* 46–61. January/February.

———. 1985b. Ensuring Entitlement to Health Care Services. *New England Economic Review* 30–40. November/December.

National Study Group on State Medicaid Strategies. 1983. *Restructuring Medicaid: An Agenda for Change*. Summary Report. Washington: Center for the Study of Social Policy.

Paringer, L. 1980. Medicare Assignment Rates of Physicians: Their Responses to Changes in Reimbursement Policy. *Health Care Financing Review* 1 (1):75–89.

Rice, T., and J. Gabel. 1986. Protecting the Elderly Against High Health Care Costs. *Health Affairs* 5 (3):6–21.

Riffer, Joyce. 1986. Physicians Say No Thanks to the Medicare Deal. *Hospitals* 60 (13):96.

Rosenwaike, I. 1985. A Demographic Portrait of the Oldest Old. *Milbank Memorial Fund Quarterly* 63 (2):187–205.

Roybal, E. R. 1986. Testimony before the Select Committee on Aging. U.S. Congress, House of Representatives. Hearing, July 30, 1985.

Savas, E. S. 1982. *Privatizing the Public Sector*. Chatham, NJ: Chatham House.

Sawyer, D., M. Ruther, A. Pagan-Berlucchi et al. 1983. *The Medicare and Medicaid Data Book, 1983*. U.S. Department of Health and Human Services, Health Care Financing Administration, Office of Research and Demonstrations. HCFA Pub. No. 03156.

Siu, A. L., F. A. Sonnenberg, W. G. Manning et al. 1986. Inappropriate Use of Hospitals in a Randomized Trial of Health Insurance Plans. *New England Journal of Medicine* 315 (20):1259–66.

Soldo, B. J., and K. G. Manton. 1985. Changes in the Health Status and Service Needs of the Oldest Old: Current Patterns and Future Trends. *Milbank Memorial Fund Quarterly* 63 (2):286–323.

Thompson, Frank J. 1981. *Health Policy and the Bureaucracy: Politics and Implementation.* Cambridge: MIT Press.

U.S. Congress House. Select Committee on Aging. 1985. *Twentieth Anniversary of Medicare and Medicaid: Americans Still at Risk.* 99th Congress, 1st session. Hearing.

U.S. Congress. Senate. Special Committee on Aging. 1984. *Medicare and the Health Costs of Older Americans: The Extent and Effects of Cost Sharing.* 98th Congress, 2d session.

U.S. Congressional Budget Office. 1983. *Changing the Structure of Medicare Benefits: Issues and Options.*

———. 1986. *Physician Reimbursement Under Medicare: Options for Change.*

U.S. Department of Health, Education and Welfare. Social Security Administration. Office of Research and Statistics. 1973. *Current Medicare Survey Report: Impact of Cost-Sharing on Use of Ambulatory Services Under Medicare: Preliminary Findings, 1969.* DHEW Pub. No. (SSA)74-11702.

U.S. Department of Health and Human Services. 1984. *Annual Medicare Program Statistics.* HCFA Pub. No. 03189.

———. 1985. *Analysis of State Medicaid Program Characteristics, 1984.* Health Care Financing Administration Publication No. 03204. Baltimore, MD.

U.S. Department of Labor. Bureau of Labor Statistics. 1985. *Consumer Expenditure Survey: Interview Survey, 1980–81.* Bulletin 2225.

Vladeck, B. C., and J. P. Firman. 1983. The Aging of the Population and Health Services. *Annals, AAPSS* 468:132–48. July.

Waldo, D. R., and H. C. Lazenby. 1984. Demographic Characteristics and Health Care Use and Expenditures by the Aged in the United States: 1977–1984. *Health Care Financing Review* 6 (1):1–29.

Waldo, D. R., K. R. Levit and H. Lazenby. 1986. National Health Expenditures, 1985. *Health Care Financing Review* 8 (1):1–21.

Wan, T. T. H. 1982. Use of Health Services by the Elderly in Low-Income Communities. *Milbank Memorial Fund Quarterly* 60 (1):82–107.

Wetle, T. 1985. Future Society's Outlook Toward Aging, Illness, and Health Care of the Aged. In *Aging 2000: Our Health Care Destiny.* Volume II: *Psychosocial and Policy Issues,* ed. C. M. Gaitz, G. Niederehe and N. L. Wilson. New York: Springer-Verlag.

4

Medicare's Coverage of Health Services

MARK SCHLESINGER
TERRIE WETLE

Much of what happens in Washington is shaped by the political mores and taboos that constitute the conventional wisdom of the day. One of the most powerful involves "not fiddling with a popular program." Proposals to change such programs are strongly resisted for fear of disrupting the political coalition that provides support. Such programs assume a sort of political sanctity, placing them outside the normal political process that leads to incremental reform. If, however, reforms are necessary to adapt the program to a changing environment, this reticence to change may leave the program progressively less effective, sapping the very political support that opponents of change have sought to preserve.

In our assessment, this is exactly what is happening to Medicare's provisions covering health care services. In an effort to preserve a politically popular program, the services covered by Medicare have been left much as they were when the legislation was drafted. Much outside the program, though, has changed in the past two decades. The private insurance policies on which Medicare was modeled in 1965 offered much narrower coverage than is available to most working Americans today. The average age of Medicare beneficiaries has increased considerably between 1965 and 1987, resulting in different health care needs. Moreover, our understanding of those needs is more complete now than it was some twenty years ago. The health care system itself has changed, creating different problems for elder patients.

If the Medicare program is to serve its beneficiaries as well in the future as it has in the past, it must adapt to these ongoing changes. It has not. And by remaining unchanged, it has exacerbated problems confronting the elderly. Unable to obtain coverage for needed services under Medicare's auspices, the elderly are forced to turn to Medicaid and private supplementary insurance policies. The resulting array of coverages has led to a confusing and fragmented system in which, all too often, elders fail to receive timely and appropriate care.

In this chapter, we identify the limitations of Medicare's current service coverage and examine the forces that have hampered past efforts to modify the program to meet changing needs. We review major proposals in light of these inhibiting factors, seeking reforms that enable Medicare to better serve the elderly.

Changing Needs and an Unchanging Program

Current Coverage and Its Origins

One of the strongest political arguments favoring Medicare's initial passage was equity—that the elderly should have access, at reasonable cost, to the types of health insurance coverage available to working Americans. It is not surprising, then, that Medicare's coverage of services was designed to be very much like that available to employee groups through commercial insurers. In fact, Part B was modeled on health insurance available to federal employees through the Aetna Insurance Company (Marmor, 1970).

In Medicare's hurried enactment, little thought was given to whether the services covered by these policies were appropriate for the elderly. Almost all of the debate on coverage centered on whether there would be financial limits on benefits and, if so, what these would be. What emerged from the House-Senate conference committee in July 1965 was a program that provided principally for the costs of treating acute illnesses.

Hospital coverage was defined in terms of benefit periods, each beginning with a hospitalization and ending 60 days after discharge. After the payment of a deductible, Medicare was to fully pay for 60 days of care in each benefit period. An additional 30 days of coverage was available if the beneficiary paid a 25 percent copayment. Eighty percent of all inpatient physician care was covered after payment of a small deductible.

Care outside the general hospital was less comprehensively covered. Nursing home services were limited exclusively to rehabilitation from an acute illness, and then only for up to 100 days per benefit period. To enforce this restriction nursing home coverage was available only after a stay in the hospital and only for services defined as "skilled nursing care." The latter requirement was particularly restrictive because many beneficiaries who required institutional care did not need the intensity of care established as "skilled." Because of these restrictions, far less than 100 days of effective coverage was actually available to the average enrollee. Not surprisingly, the average length of a Medicare-covered stay was only about 16 days. Care in psychiatric hospitals was also covered but with a 190-day-lifetime ceiling.

Coverage of outpatient services incorporated additional restrictions. Eighty percent of "reasonable" physicians' charges were covered, but neither regular physical exams nor prescription drugs were included. Outpatient mental health care was paid for only up to $500 a year with a 50 percent copayment required. Home health care was covered for one hundred visits a year, but only for elders who were homebound and in need of skilled nursing care. Like most private insurance during this period, Medicare did not cover dental care, hearing aids or eyeglasses.

In the subsequent two decades, Medicare benefits were changed from time to time. For the most part, changes involved expansions or contractions of services already defined as reimbursable rather than changes in the scope of coverage. An additional 60-day "life-time reserve" of hospital coverage was added, though a 50 percent copayment was built into this coverage. A few specialty services, such as podiatry, were included under coverage of physician's services. More recently, requirements for prior hospitalization for home health and nursing home coverage were eliminated as was the limit on the number of home health visits covered. These liberalizations were to some extent offset, however, by more restrictive administrative interpretations of the "skilled nursing care" requirement for home health care (Feder and Scanlon, 1982; National Association of Home Care, 1986).

The only significant expansion in coverage designed to meet the needs of elder beneficiaries occurred 17 years after the program was enacted[1] In 1982, as part of the Tax Equity and Fiscal Responsibility Act (TEFRA), Congress extended Medicare coverage to hospice care, a set of special services for patients with terminal diseases. Even this extension involved, in large part, services already covered by the program (Dunlop, 1983). Nonetheless, the willingness to incorporate this new service represented an important exception to a history of largely unchanging coverage. We will, therefore, explore the circumstances surrounding this reform in some detail later in this chapter.

Changing Standards for Medicare Coverage

Although Medicare's coverage provisions have remained largely unchanged, much outside the program has changed dramatically. Three changes in particular have altered the standards by which we judge Medicare's coverage of services: (1) changes in private insurance coverage for younger Americans, (2) changes in our understanding of the health needs of the elderly, and (3) changes in the types of services required by older persons.

Slipping Out of the Mainstream

As noted, Medicare was modeled on the insurance coverage available to the working-age population in 1965. This was intended to bring elders into the mainstream of American health care. By the 1980s, however, private plans had expanded their coverage to a far broader range of services.

- In 1965, less than 5 percent of the privately insured were covered for dental care. By 1981, over half had dental insurance (Health Insurance Association of America, 1983).
- Medicare's $250-a-year coverage of outpatient mental health care was fairly generous by 1965 standards but has not increased despite high inflation of health care costs. By the mid-1980s, 10 percent of privately insured people working in major corporations had no dollar limitation on outpatient coverage of mental health care; almost 70 percent had over $1,500 a year in coverage (Muszynski et al., 1983).
- In 1965, few private insurance policies covered the costs of prescription drugs. In 1984, more than a quarter of these costs were paid through private insurance (Levit, et al., 1985).

Medicare, though, continues to emulate coverages from over twenty years in the past; caught in an eddy, its beneficiaries have drifted out of the mainstream. As a result, the elderly's access to certain health care services has suffered when compared with younger Americans.

There are a number of disturbing consequences. The elderly have a far higher rate of untreated dental problems than do younger Americans (Pegels, 1980), yet those over the age of 65 are twice as likely as other adults to have gone two years without seeing a dentist (U.S. Department of Health and Human Services, 1984). Recent surveys have shown that the elderly are twice as likely to have untreated mental illness as are middle-aged individuals in the same community (Shapiro et al, 1985).

Changing Understanding of Elders' Needs

In borrowing coverage provisions from insurance policies of younger Americans, Medicare's designers implicitly assumed that elders' health care needs were very much like those of their younger counterparts. We now understand that this assumption is incorrect. Elders have certain special needs that merit coverage different from that offered by private insurance.

First, elders are more likely to suffer from chronic illness than are younger age groups. The average 70-year-old has twice as many days of restricted activity owing to chronic conditions as does the typical 40-year-old (Butler and Newacheck, 1981). By failing to cover the treatment of chronic illness in nursing homes and home health care agencies, Medicare overlooks important needs of its beneficiaries. This leads to untreated illness and substantial financial burdens. For example, it has been estimated that a 13-week stay in a nursing home would impoverish over half of all elders (U.S Congress, House, Select Committee on Aging, 1985).

Second, the health care needs of the elderly are more difficult for physicians to assess than those of younger patients. Elder patients typically have multiple illnesses—the average hospitalized elder has six pathological conditions—and many diseases present symptoms uncommon in younger patients and thus unfamiliar to many doctors (Besdine, 1982; Rowe, 1985). These problems are complicated by the complex interactions of health, economic and social needs in the elderly, factors that many physicians find uninteresting or difficult to assess (Rowe, 1985; U.S. General Accounting Office, 1979).

To promote more accurate evaluation of older patients it has been suggested that nonphysicians play a larger role in the assessment process. A report from the Inspector General's Office in the Department of Health and Human Services (DHHS), for example, recommended that "nurses and social workers must become more clearly and officially accountable for client assessment and case management functions. This is important . . . to help clients obtain the package of services that will maximize their opportunity for functional independence" (Monier et al., 1981, p. 10). Under current coverage provisions, Medicare does nothing to encourage such interdisciplinary geriatric assessments. In fact, it tends to discourage innovative approaches that use providers other than physicians by requiring that virtually all reimbursable services be provided under the direct supervision of a physician.

Third, elders often lack the information they need to effectively plan for and use health services. This stems in part from the fact that elders need both medical and social services to meet their chronic and acute health needs and the system that delivers those services is fragmented into literally hundreds of programs and agencies (Callahan, 1981; Morris and Youket, 1981.)

Confusion also occurs because elders must deal with a complex health system and Medicare program without the help supplied to younger Americans when they purchase insurance or use health care services. Books designed to explain Medicare benefits typically contain more than three hundred pages of fine print and are filled with so many contingency clauses and exceptions that they would be confusing to any reader. Beneficiaries must try to understand these complicated provisions without the advice of the benefits managers available to most of those who have insurance through employer groups (Firman, 1985).[2]

To address these problems, the elderly must be provided with information and offered assistance in selecting needed services. Unfortunately, Medicare does not pay for these informational services. In the words of a nurse working in a home health agency, "The problem is there's no reimbursement for case management. Since it's expensive and time consuming, no one really does it" (Inspector General, 1981, p. 10).

As a result, needed services go unused or are inappropriately used. A 1979 study by the General Accounting Office (GAO) found, for example, that between 50 and 80 percent of the elderly did not know about home health care services available in their community. Many elders do not even know how information about such services can be obtained (Holmes et al., 1983). Services that *are* used are often poorly matched to elders' health care needs. Past studies indicate that between 20 and 50 percent of the elders in nursing homes were inappropriately placed in those institutions (Winn and McCaffree, 1979).

Changing Needs of the Elderly

The inadequacies of Medicare's coverage have been exacerbated over the past two decades by changes in the health care requirements of the elderly and increases in elders' need for reliable sources of information. The strongest determinant of changing needs has been the rising average age of the population covered by Medicare. In 1960, less than 5 percent of the Medicare population was older than 85. By 1985, the proportion of Medicare beneficiaries over the age of 85 had doubled; by the year 2050, it is predicted that a quarter of all beneficiaries will be 85 or older (Rosenwaike, 1985).

With advanced age comes a marked increase in the prevalence of chronic illness and the need for long-term services. Beneficiaries over 85 are 15 times more likely to be admitted to a nursing home than those between the ages of 65 and 74 (Butler and Newacheck, 1981). Older beneficiaries are far more likely to require daily support services to continue to live at home (Soldo and Manton, 1985). As the Medicare population continues to age over the next 50 years, the program's current benefits—oriented as they are toward acute care—will become less and less adequate to meet the health care requirements of the nation's elders.

Beneficiaries also have greater need for reliable sources of information as a result of the increasing complexity of the Medicare program. Enrollees today must choose between the traditional program and alternative coverages through Medicare-affiliated health maintenance organizations (HMOs) (Iglehart, 1985). They also face choices between traditional providers and newly emerging emergency medical centers, walk-in clinics and other innovative arrangements. Without additional information and assistance, many beneficiaries may be unable to choose wisely when faced with these complex decisions (lFirman, 1985; Greenfield, 1986).

At the same time that the Medicare program and the health care system are becoming more complex, reliable sources of information are disappearing. Historically, elders have relied on hospital discharge planners to help arrange for needed services (Inspector General, 1981). When Medicare switched to prospective payment of hospitals in 1983, however, the reimbursement system created incentives for early discharge of patients. Under these conditions, beneficiaries have increasingly feared that the interests of the hospital no longer coincide with their own welfare and thus are less trusting of advice from these traditional sources (Kerschner, 1986).

With few changes in coverage over the past two decades, the Medicare program has thus fallen behind private insurers and is less able to meet the needs of its beneficiaries. The full effect of these shortcomings can be understood, however, only by reviewing the alternatives to which elders turned in seeking more adequate coverage.

The Patchwork Insurance Coverage of the Elderly

With Medicare's evident limitations, beneficiaries have been forced to look elsewhere to help pay for needed medical services. For protection from the costs of long-term care, they have turned to the Medicaid program. In response to other coverage limits, they have purchased private insurance, typically termed supplementary, or Medigap, policies. Each of these alternatives has its own shortcomings. Moreover, the combination of Medicare, Medicaid and Medigap leaves many elders caught in a complex, yet inadequate, web of policies, payment schemes and paperwork.

Medicaid and the Coverage of Long-term Care

Medicaid was passed as companion legislation to the Medicare program. It was intended in part to provide additional financial protection for the elderly who are poor or medically indigent, that is, those whose incomes were sufficiently limited that medical expenses might cause major financial hardship. Ironically, Medicaid's strongest proponents were conservative legislators who hoped it would forestall efforts to expand Medicare or create a national health insurance system.

Medicaid was not intended to be a primary means of paying for long-term care. However, because nursing home costs are so large, paying for care soon reduces most elders' assets to the point that they become Medicaid-eligible. As a result, Medicaid inadvertently became the principal form of public payment of nursing home care in this country. As of 1984, Medicaid paid $14 billion for nursing home care, 45 percent of total national spending in these facilities.

Medicaid thus represents an important source of financial support for the chronically ill elderly. As a program of financing for long-term care, however, Medicaid is haphazardly structured and incomplete. "Medicaid, hastily enacted and created, was only a sideshow in the health insurance circus. Decisions had been made serially, one at a time: first nursing home coverage under Medicare was limited; then Medicaid was added to Medicare; then nursing homes were included under Medicaid—and then the process stopped" (Vladeck, 1980, p. 51). As a result of many of the hurried decisions embodied in the legislation, Medicaid became a program that to many elders seems unreliable and, to many more, unacceptable.

The lack of reliability stems from Medicaid's basic structure. It is a program of collaboration between state and federal governments. In this collaboration, states are given wide discretion in establishing eligibility standards, coverage provisions and reimbursement arrangements for the program. As a result:

- There is tremendous interstate variation in standards for eligibility. The proportion of the poor elderly covered in the most generous states is ten times as large as in the least generous; in 10 states, less than a third of all elders with incomes below the poverty line are covered by Medicaid (U.S. General Accounting Office, 1979).
- Even when eligible, elders in some states are covered for a far-more-limited array of services than in others. The most generous states cover 3 times as many optional services as the least generous (Davidson and Marmor, 1980).
- Even when eligible and covered, beneficiaries often have difficulty obtaining care because the Medicaid program pays providers at rates so low that they may refuse to treat the patients (U.S. General Accounting Office, 1979; Brecher and Knickman, 1985). One study conducted in Massachusetts in 1976 found that Medicaid enrollees waited up to 16 times longer to be admitted to a nursing home than did comparable patients who paid for their own care (Gruenberg and Willemain, 1982).

Medicaid coverage is perceived by many elders as unacceptable for two reasons. First, the program creates financial incentives for beneficiaries to become institutionalized. Even in the most generous states—with the possible exception of New York—the long-term-care services that Medicaid covers favor institutional care (Morris and Youket, 1981; Rosenfeld, 1982). This reinforces a bias created by eligibility requirements. Many elders with moderate incomes cannot qualify for Medicaid benefits; therefore they cannot obtain coverage of home health care and are then forced into a nursing home. Once institutionalized, they rapidly exhaust their financial resources, qualifying for Medicaid, but at that point their health or financial status no longer allows them to return to the community (Davis and Rowland, 1986).

Elders also find Medicaid unacceptable because to qualify for coverage they are required in many states to impoverish themselves and their households. Rather than provide security for older Americans, this demeans them. For example, in New York one spouse is sometimes forced to sue the other for support while he or she is in an institution. Such a situation was described in a recent newspaper article:

> After 51 years of marriage, Morris and Bertha Hafner could not believe that their modest lives together would ever come to this: that she would be forced to sue him for support while he lay helpless in a Bronx nursing home. 'It's cruel and humiliating,' Mrs. Hafner said the other day with tears in her eyes. 'It's not right,' she said. 'Older people should not be humiliated and made to suffer like this' (*New York Times*, March 6, 1986, p. 1).

To avoid such humiliation, many elders will refuse Medicaid's services for which they are eligible. A recent poll by the American Association of Retired Persons

(AARP) found that 40 percent of elderly were reluctant to seek Medicaid eligibility (Sokoloff and Sota, 1985). When elders refuse to make use of Medicaid, even in the face of tremendous financial hardships, serious questions are raised about the overall effectiveness of current arrangements for paying for long-term care.

Medicare's Limitations and Medigap Policies

Given the limitations and uncertainties in public coverage, it is not surprising that elders have turned to private insurance. Over two thirds of Medicare's beneficiaries have purchased these so-called Medigap policies (Hagen, 1986). Such policies do add to Medicare's coverage to some extent. Roughly 60 percent of the policies pay for some mental health care, 40 percent for some of the costs of out-of-hospital prescription drugs, and about 4 percent provide some form of dental coverage (Cafferata, 1984b).

Nonetheless, for the most part, these private policies incorporate the very same restrictions as does Medicare (Feder and Holahan, 1979). "Private insurance purchased by the elderly is generally oriented to the services covered by Medicare . . . private insurance for services excluded from Medicare benefits [is] held by relatively few" (Cafferata, 1984b, p. 8). Unfortunately, many of the elders purchasing policies do not recognize these limitations. Fully 50 percent expect their insurance to pay a substantial share of nursing home expenses, though virtually none, in fact, do so (Hagen, 1986). Many erroneously believe that Medigap policies will cover other forms of long-term care as well (Meiners, 1983; Sokoloff and Sota, 1985).

This misunderstanding occurs in part because supplementary policies are complicated, with many exclusions and detailed limitations (Firman, 1985). In some cases, these policies have also been marketed in a deceptive manner (Inspector General, 1981). A study by the Federal Trade Commission (FTC) in the 1970s found that a quarter of all elders had purchased supplementary policies that were essentially worthless because they simply duplicated coverage provided by Medicare or by another private policy (Pegels, 1980). Although the federal government and many states have attempted to regulate insurance practices, there is no clear evidence that these regulations have been successfully enforced, and anecdotal accounts suggest that at least some fraudulent marketing practices continue (Hagen, 1986).

Many private policies also have very high administrative expenses. During the 1970s, it was not unusual to find policies that paid out as little as 20 percent of their premiums in the form of benefits (Feder and Holahan, 1979). Since then, federal and state regulations have sought to prohibit the sale of policies with low returns to beneficiaries. Beginning in 1982, the Baucus amendment to the Social Security Act required that policies labeled "Medicare Supplementary Policies" pay out at least 60 percent of their premiums in benefits. It remains to be seen whether this regulation will be successfully enforced; plans that go under other names, even if sold to the elderly for the purpose of complementing Medicare coverage, are exempted from the legislation. Even if the regulation is effective, the administrative and marketing costs of such policies remain high compared to the administrative costs of the Medicare program, which in 1984 were less than 3 percent of total program spending (Levit et al., 1985).

Finally, because private policies are purchased on a voluntary basis, they run the risk of what economists term adverse selection. Individuals who have the highest risk of needing a particular service are most likely to purchase coverage of that service. This limits the ability of the insurance company to spread risks, and may make the cost of private policies quite high, particularly for those policies that focus on specific services (Feder and Holahan, 1979; Bishop, 1981).

To limit the risk of adverse selection, insurers often attempt to selectively market to low-risk groups (Meiners, 1983). This holds down premiums for these groups but makes insurance that is available to all elders more expensive. Alternatively, plans may impose a complex set of restrictions on coverage designed to screen out the high-risk enrollee (Piktialis, 1986). These restrictions further limit the availability and breadth of private insurance for many elders.

Elders' Problems with Patchwork Insurance Coverage

Whatever the individual limitations of Medicare, Medicaid and Medigap plans, there are clearly some advantages to a system that combines the three sets of coverage. In certain states Medicaid provides comprehensive coverage for the poor elderly. Some Medicaid programs pay for visits to an optometrist, the cost of eyeglasses, dental care, prescription drugs and diagnostic examinations. Because these services are limited to those with low incomes, public programs can afford to be more generous to those most in need.

Using private insurance to selectively broaden insurance coverage also has some advantages. Not all elders prefer the same types of coverage. Allowing individuals to select the private policy that they believe best fits their needs and concerns introduces flexibility that would be difficult to achieve in a uniform public insurance program.

Nonetheless, the limitations of this patchwork system are real and, under many circumstances, outweigh its advantages. The current system creates tremendous inequities. Elders in states with generous Medicaid programs do far better than their counterparts in other states. Those who do not qualify for, or refuse to use, Medicaid are forced to pay for the potentially catastrophic costs of long-term care from their own resources. Elders are driven to purchase expensive private insurance policies in an almost desperate—and largely fruitless—effort to avoid exposure to potentially impoverishing financial burdens.

Some of the greatest shortcomings of the current system, however, are created not by the individual limitations of Medicare, Medicaid or Medigap plans but by the interaction of all three together. At the very least, this array of coverages vastly complicates elders' task of making sense of their insurance arrangements. Faced by three (or more, if they own several private policies) different sets of coverages, restrictions and eligibility requirements, elders are less likely to fully understand any single plan. Beneficiaries may fail to use care for which they are covered or fail to file for and receive reimbursement for the care received (Feder and Holahan, 1979).[3]

The current patchwork system also leads to higher costs in several ways. Policies tend to inadvertantly subsidize one another, leading to the purchase of an excessive amount of insurance. For example, many Medigap policies pay for the copayments built into the Medicare program. In so doing, they remove the financial incentive to use health care prudently and thus increase the overall costs of the health care system. Most of these extra costs, though, are paid for by the Medicare program. Medicare is thus indirectly subsidizing about 30 percent of the value of private plans that do not bear the full cost of the health care use they stimulate (Ginsburg, 1983). As a result, these plans can be sold at lower cost, thus encouraging more elders to purchase insurance and further promoting utilization.

The current mix of coverages also inhibits attempts to reduce costs. It is often suggested that more effective management of patient care could reduce inappropriate utilization (Inspector General, 1981; Somers, 1982). But case management is complicated because many elders begin to use care while paying in one way, then later shift to another source of financing.

For example, 44 states have incorporated into their Medicaid programs some form of screening to limit inappropriate institutionalization in nursing homes (Hekman, 1984). Screening can be effective, however, only when elders' needs are assessed before they enter a nursing home. Once in a facility for an extended period, many elders develop physical or psychological dependencies that make discharge difficult; others have been forced to sell their homes or give up their apartments and thus have no place in the community to which they can return (Inspector General, 1981). The majority of elders admitted to a nursing home pay for care from private resources; only after they have been institutionalized for a time do they spend down to Medicaid eligibility. They thus inadvertently bypass the screening and case-management systems built into Medicaid programs.[4]

Finally, the current mix of coverages leads to poorer quality health care. In some cases, patients may be bounced from one provider to another as they exhaust one form of insurance benefit and move to another coverage that reimburses care only in particular settings (Cuccaro, 1980).[5] In other cases, patients are transferred from one facility to another to qualify for coverage of specific illnesses. For example, a mentally ill Medicaid eligible nursing home resident may be discharged to a hospital so that Medicare will pay for the psychiatric care that Medicaid did not adequately cover. This shifting disrupts continuity of care and probably, in itself, harms the health of elders (Pegels, 1980).

Perhaps equally important, in the current system, no single payer is responsible for the full array of health services used by the elderly. When elders encounter gaps in the service system or unfair treatment, they may be unable to determine where to turn for recourse (Firman, 1985).

For all these reasons, there is growing dissatisfaction with current arrangements for insuring against the costs of elders' health care needs. Medicare's coverage is viewed as too narrow and inflexible, Medicaid's as inequitable and unacceptable, and Medigap plans as incomplete and overly expensive. The entire patchwork array seems frayed. To address these shortcomings reforms could—and undoubtedly should—be made in each of these three sets of coverage. We focus here on proposed reforms of the Medicare program.

Prospects and Options for Change in Medicare's Coverage

By failing to adapt to changing standards of coverage and needs of the elderly, Medicare's coverage has become less adequate to meet the requirements of its beneficiaries. A number of proposals have been advanced that would address these inadequacies by adding coverage to improve both long-term and primary care of older patients. Though each of these proposals has some appeal, whether they will prove desirable or feasible depends to a large extent on their ability to address certain issues. These constraints on change can best be understood by reviewing the historical factors that have inhibited reform in the past.

Historical Constraints on Coverage Reform

As with any public program, Medicare has been shaped by a number of political and social forces. It is therefore difficult to determine exactly which have been most responsible for the stasis in Medicare's coverage provisions in the face of their growing inadequacies. In our assessment, however, Medicare's failure to adapt to changing conditions can be largely attributed to three factors: (1) the image of the program created in congressional debate surrounding Medicare's enactment, (2) the program's early experience in covering services that involved chronic illnesses, and (3) the political stance taken by elder Americans and their advocates.

The prolonged political debate in the decade preceding Medicare's enactment and the flurry of negotiation accompanying its legislative passage did much to shape the thinking of Congress—as well as the rest of the country—about the appropriate role for the Medicare program in the American health care system. In so doing, certain types of reform were made to seem politically risky, potentially disrupting the coalition of interests that emerged in support of the program. More subtly, the debate created a particular image for the Medicare program and linked it with certain goals, implicitly setting other objectives outside the bounds of political discourse.

As noted in Chapter 1, organized medicine had passionately and publicly opposed the legislation creating Medicare. Even after Medicare's enactment was assured, there were concerns that doctors and hospitals might boycott the program, making it impossible for beneficiaries to gain access to care (Feder, 1977). Hence, the Johnson administration and proponents of the program in Congress took great care to tailor the legislation as much as possible to meet the interests of providers. As a result, "the very medical providers who had so bitterly fought the legislation now faced a statute dripping with incentives for them to cooperate" (Thompson, 1981, p. 160).

These incentives took several forms. To guarantee that Medicare would not create competitors to existing physicians and hospitals, Congress gave substantial control over Medicare's accreditation process to those providers and agreed not to reimburse other providers who might compete for patients. For example, Medicare reimbursed only those ambulatory services approved by a physician, so that other service providers could be paid only at a physician's discretion. Perhaps most telling was Section 1801 of the law. Titled "Prohibition Against any Federal Interference," this section prohibited the government from exerting "any supervision or control over . . . the manner in which medical services are provided."

By structuring the legislation in this way, Congress limited the ability of Medicare to adapt to the changing needs of its beneficiaries. By prohibiting interference, the legislation limited the program's ability to stimulate changes in the delivery system that might promote the health of older patients. Even apart from this legal constraint, the program had been structured in a way that made it unresponsive to many unmet needs. Appropriateness of services was defined almost exclusively in narrow, medical terms. Medical treatments alone are often insufficient to meet the health needs of the elderly, and a program modeled in the interests of physicians tends to be insensitive to these shortcomings.

Medicare beneficiaries also became the victims of a broader political debate surrounding the enactment of the program in 1965. Conservatives feared that Medicare was the first step in a political march toward universal public health insurance. To prevent this, they engineered a far more generous Medicare program than that proposed by the Kennedy and Johnson administrations, one that Congress and the public would perceive as not requiring subsequent expansion. The intention was to politically "build a fence" around the Medicare program (Marmor, 1969).

This fence was intended to keep out national health insurance, but it also served to limit the scope of Medicare's benefits by creating the impression that the program was already sufficiently comprehensive. Over the years, as prospects for national health insurance receded and the political atmosphere became more hostile toward new federal expenditures, Medicare's advocates focused on preserving rather than improving the program. They regarded proposals for significant reform as "politically unfeasible," prefering to make "minor cosmetic adjustments that we can rationalize as 'preserving the integrity of the program' rather than confront the failure and success of the program as it functions in a contemporary context" (Binstock, 1985, p. 428).

The second reason that Medicare's coverage provisions have proven so inflexible stems from early program experience with services involving chronic illnesses. In several instances, these services proved unexpectedly expensive, raising the fear that any expanded coverage of services for chronic illness would lead to uncontrollable growth in program costs.

The first such episode occurred shortly after the program was passed. Although Medicare's nursing-home- and home-health-care provisions were intended to pay only for rehabilitation from acute illnesses, the Social Security Administration's initial definitions were sufficiently vague that providers applied for reimbursement for treatment of a much broader group of patients, including many with chronic diseases. Partially as a result, costs of these coverages greatly exceeded projections made when the legislation was passed. By 1967, nursing home coverage was six to seven times as costly as expected, home health care two to three times as expensive (U.S. Congress, Senate, Committee on Finance, 1970).

Federal officials responded by hastily rewriting definitions of reimbursable services; nursing homes were retroactively denied reimbursement for care that they had already provided. Medicare spending on nursing home care fell 60 percent within one year (Feder and Scanlon, 1982). In the minds of many in Washington, however, services related to long-term care had already been linked with the specter of skyrocketing costs.

Medicare's second exposure to services directed at the chronically ill came in 1972. Amendments to the Social Security Act passed in that year made individuals with end-stage renal disease (ESRD) eligible for Medicare coverage.[6] Once again, program costs vastly exceeded initial expectations, growing from $283 million in 1974 to $1.2 billion in 1980. Most of this increase was created because many more patients were dialyzed than had been anticipated. The number of patients increased from 16,000 in 1974 to 64,000 in 1981, leading some observers to conclude that program costs were "wildly out of control" (Lowrie and Hampers, 1982, p. 191).

These two experiences left deep impressions on administrators of the Medicare program and many in Congress. Expensive programs create political concern in themselves, but the specter of *uncontrollable* expenses—particularly in the era of Gramm–Rudman—has made coverage of services for chronic illness about as popular an issue for many politicians as finding sites for storing nuclear waste. Many recognize the need, but few want to pay the price of finding an acceptable solution. Because many of the unmet needs of Medicare's beneficiaries involve chronic illness, this concern hangs over almost any proposal to reform Medicare's coverage of health care services.

The final factor discouraging expansion of Medicare's coverage has been the political stance of the elderly. Elder interest groups have been vociferous in resisting cuts in Medicare benefits but much less active in encouraging expansion. This is probably due, in part, to a misperception about the breadth of current coverage. Almost 80 percent of the elderly believe that Medicare would pay for an extended stay in a nursing home. Two thirds of the elderly do not understand the limitations on Medicare's coverage of home health and mental health care (Lambert, 1980; Cafferata, 1984a). With such widespread misunderstanding, mobilizing political support for changes in coverage is difficult.

In addition, elder groups are concerned that advocating reform in financing and eligibility would raise basic and difficult questions about the mission and direction of the program. Much of the political support for the enactment of Medicare came not simply because it would improve the health of the elderly, but because the elderly as a group had severely limited financial resources (Bayer and Callahan, 1985). "Since the early 1960s, these 'advocates for the aged' have been telling us that the elderly are poor, frail, socially dependent, objects of discrimination and, above all, *deserving*. . . . Because older persons came to be stereotyped as 'the deserving poor' they have been exempted from the Calvinist screenings that are applied to other Americans in order to determine whether they are worthy of public assistance" (Binstock, 1985, p. 429).

Since 1965, however, the financial status of America's elders has changed. The poverty rate among those over 65 is now virtually identical to those under 65. This raises questions about whether the Medicare program should continue to subsidize insurance coverage for all elders—poor and nonpoor alike—to the same extent. Redirecting Medicare benefits to elders with less income, though, raises concerns that Medicare would become viewed as a welfare program and that programs for the poor become poor programs. Consequently, for many Medicare supporters, preserving the program, even with its flawed coverage provisions, appears preferable to reopening debate over its fundamental goals.

Taken together, these three broad factors—the image of the program created in the initial legislative debate, early program experience with services for the chronically ill, and the conservative political stance of America's elderly toward program reform—have combined to limit change in Medicare's coverage provisions over the past 20-plus years. These are not, however, insurmountable barriers to change. Some coverages, including ESRD and hospice provisions, have been added to the program. The constraints themselves can change over time; Medicare's adoption of diagnostic-related groups (DRGs) represented a shift away from noninterference, being explicitly intended to change the behavior of health care providers (see Chapter 5). Institutional innovations may also circumvent constraints of the past. The high costs associated with paying for chronic illness occurred under fee-for-service reimbursements, with treatment left to the discretion of providers. New methods of paying and organizing services (through prepayment and case management) may offer ways to extend coverage without creating uncontrollable increases in costs.

Historical factors do, however, define an implicit set of criteria that proposals must pass if further reform is to be feasible. Identifying these will help to better assess the prospects for specific reform proposals.

Prospects for Reform

Medicare's history suggests three criteria for successful future reform. First, any proposal must gain the support of both beneficiaries and younger taxpayers. To achieve broad-based support among younger Americans, it must be demonstrated that the service meets needs vital to the well-being of beneficiaries. To capture beneficiaries' support, a plan must not simply meet the needs of the elderly; it must also address issues that can galvanize elders to work actively for change.

Past expansions of coverage, for both ESRD and hospice care, touched on issues of life and death and thus had great political saliency. Vance Hartke, (1972) sponsor of the ESRD amendments, cogently expressed this salience, "In what must be the most tragic irony of the twentieth century, people are dying because they cannot get access to proper medical care. We have learned how to treat or to cure some diseases which have plagued mankind for centuries yet these treatments are not available to most Americans because of their costs". As the successful inclusion of hospice benefits demonstrates, expansion need not involve life-saving treatment. It does need to tap some equally powerful concern such as "death with dignity."[7]

Second, it must be demonstrated that Medicare can address current shortcomings more adequately than can either Medicaid or private supplementary policies. Because limitations in Medicare have, by default, relegated substantial coverage to other parts of the current patchwork system, both Medicaid and Medigap plans have developed a track record and a certain political legitimacy in meeting some needs. Even apart from this history, it makes sense to assign to Medicare what it can do best and resolve other problems through other mechanisms. This may involve shifting some services now covered by Medicaid to Medicare or vice versa. The current political climate, though, certainly favors both state-based reforms and private initiative (Meyer, 1983; Glenn and Brazda, 1985). Only where the private market and state programs can be shown to be inadequate will Medicare reform be seriously considered.

Third, extending Medicare coverage will be feasible only if it can be demonstrated that the resulting increases in program costs are predictable and controllable. In the era of Gramm–Rudman, there is, of course, resistance to proposals that increase program costs at all. Over the longer term, we anticipate that the potential costs of proposed reforms will be weighed in a more balanced manner against their benefits. We also predict, however, that Congress will remain sensitive to cost implications and will expand benefits only if costs clearly can be controlled. Hospice benefits were included under Medicare, for example, only with the provision that (1) each beneficiary had a limited number of days of coverage and (2) for each episode of hospice treatment, reimbursement paid to the hospice agency was "capped" so that it could not exceed a preset amount.

Options for Coverage Reform

Proposals for changing Medicare's service coverage can be grouped into a half dozen categories: (1) long-term health care, (2) case management services, (3) social support services, (4) mental health care, (5) prevention and primary care, and (6) ancillary health care expenses. We will assess each type of proposal by the three criteria identified above. In addition, specific proposals in each category sometimes differ in the approach or administrative detail. We will discuss the more important of these distinctions and consider how they affect the feasibility or desirability of proposed reforms

Long-Term Care Services

Over half the elderly suffer from some form of chronic illness (Soldo and Manton, 1985). For about a third of these individuals, chronic conditions lead to significant impairment of their daily activities (Weissert, 1985). Most of these elders continue to live at home, though about 1.5 million elders are admitted to a nursing home each year, and 20 percent of all elders will enter a nursing home at some point in their lives.

Under current arrangments, long-term-care services are fragmented and beneficiaries often are unaware of the availability of care. This places a heavy burden on the elders' family (Doty, 1986), may lead to excessive institutionalization or other inappropriate treatment (Morris and Youket, 1981) and threatens the financial security of the elderly (U.S. Congress, House, Select Committee on Aging, 1985). "Of all the difficult health-care issues facing the nation today, none is more complex or urgent than the formulation of a viable policy of long-term care for the elderly and the chronically ill and disabled. The tragic irony of the existing neglect is clearly evident in the plight of millions of frail and dependent elderly" (Somers, 1982, p. 221).

To address these problems, it has been proposed that Medicare pay for both home health and nursing home care for the chronically ill.[8] Plans differ in their details. Some simply suggest eliminating Medicare's current restriction on "custodial care" (Somers, 1982); others call for a complete redefinition of services. Some plans would make long-term-care coverage a voluntary option for beneficiaries (Davis and Rowland, 1986), others would make enrollment mandatory (Blumenthal et al., 1986).

Long-term-care services seem to meet the first two criteria for feasible reform: They are of great concern to both young and old Americans and are inadequately handled under the current patchwork array of coverages. The costs of chronic illness, particularly of care in nursing homes, represent a clear and continued threat to the emotional and financial security of older Americans. This financial threat and the link to the end of life give these services great emotional and political saliency to both elders and their children.

Alternative coverages are inadequate and are likely to remain so. Medicaid's contribution is haphazard, with large interstate variations in eligibility and services covered. Coverage remains biased toward institutional care and many programs reimburse at rates so low that providers are unwilling to accept eligible patients. Medicaid, moreover, fails to provide basic financial protection, often requiring elders to exhaust their financial resources before becoming eligible.

Although private insurance coverage for nursing home care is expanding, it too is far from adequate, in 1984, paying for less than 1 percent of the total costs of care (Levit et al., 1985). There are, moreover, good reasons for believing that private long-term-care insurance will remain limited in the future. Few individuals are willing to purchase coverage until old age makes it more likely they will need nursing home care. At that point, however, their incomes are lower and they can less afford the cost of premiums. The average 85-year-old is more than 15 times as likely to require nursing home care than the average 65-year-old but has only two-thirds the income, about $5,500 a year (Soldo and Manton, 1985; Torrey, 1985). Under these conditions those most in need of coverage often cannot afford it. For 85-year-olds, premiums for private coverage could easily exceed $1,500 a year, well over a quarter of their income (Meiners, 1984; Davis and Rowland, 1986; Lane, 1986).

Faced with these potentially large premiums, many elders will avoid purchasing policies unless they feel an imminent need for long-term care services. This "adverse selection" will further increase the cost of insurance premiums, because insurers will be selling policies primarily to elders most likely to use services. As a consequence, insurers will be less able to spread risk across the insured population. Adverse selection can be a problem with all forms of health insurance (Pauly, 1986). It is particularly problematic for long-term care policies for several reasons.

First, for most acute illnesses, being sick in one year does not increase the odds of being ill the next. It is thus difficult for someone to determine when they are likely to need health care in the next year and to only buy insurance in advance of these costs. In contrast, once elders begin to lose their ability to function independently, they can anticipate their future need for long-term care services, and purchase policies to pay for these services.

Second, insurers can limit the problems caused by adverse selection for acute illness by not paying for conditions that existed prior to the time the beneficiary purchased the policy. It may be very difficult, however, for insurers to document past losses of functional independence. Consequently, it will prove difficult to invoke "prior condition" clauses for long-term care policies, placing insurers at greater risk for the increased costs created by adverse selection.

In addition, because insurers fear that many elders would unnecessarily substitute home health services for informal family care—resulting in prohibitively high costs—most do not offer home care coverage or do so at prices affordable only to a few (Sokoloff and Sota, 1985; Piktialis, 1986).[9] Finally, the costs of administering and marketing private insurance policies can add significantly—40 to 50 percent for individual policies—to what are already large premiums.

Estimates suggest that somewhere between one third and two thirds of the elderly could potentially afford to purchase private coverage limited solely to nursing home care (Meiners, 1983; Piktialis, 1986). Private insurance with broader coverage, including home health care, would clearly be beyond the financial means of most elders. Thus, even with the most optimistic forecasts, private insurance coverage of the costs of long-term care in the early 1990s is likely to be as inadequately developed as was elders' insurance for hospital and physician care prior to the passage of Medicare in the early 1960s. Some form of insurance will be purchased by a portion—perhaps up to a third—of the elderly population. But most elders will be unable to afford coverage, and much of the coverage that is purchased will be inadequate to provide access to an appropriate array of services.

Medicare coverage of long-term care has marked advantages over that of both Medicaid and commercial plans. Eligibility and coverage could be made uniform nationwide. Integrating long-term care with other health services would eliminate the stigma now associated with Medicaid. Costs could be spread over the entire beneficiary population—and, through the payroll tax, to younger generation—making premiums affordable to the average elder. Coverage of home health care could be integrated into that which is already a part of Medicare, reducing costs and improving coordination of services. Administrative and marketing costs would be substantially less expensive, perhaps a tenth that of private plans.

The fundamental uncertainty surrounding Medicare's coverage of long-term care involves the controllability of costs. Even proponents of extended coverage sometimes fear that the program will discover users "coming out of the woodwork" (Inspector General, 1981, p. 10). In fact, it is very likely that long-term care costs will increase once covered by Medicare. It has been estimated that the costs of Medicare's covering home health care, nursing home care and outpatient mental health care would be about $50 billion by the year 2000, an increase of roughly 40 percent over what those costs would have been in the absence of Medicare coverage (Blumenthal et al., 1986).

These cost increases, while sizable, are not uncontrollable. Several Canadian provinces provide public insurance for long-term care. Their experience suggests that after an initial increase, expenditures tend to be relatively stable, "As long-term care benefits have been introduced over the past decade in various provinces, the rate of health care spending, expressed as a proportion of the gross national product, has remained below that in the United States. . . . Despite fears in this country that expanded home care benefits might lead to runaway use, the Canadian experience shows a consistent pattern of demand leveling off after about three years." (Kane and Kane, 1985, pp. 1362–63). The ability to control costs in this manner may be related to the use of case managers in the Canadian system (Somers, 1982).

Though the costs of covering long-term care may be ultimately controllable, two related concerns remain. First, projected expenditures are so large that even relatively minor cost overruns may place large burdens on the federal budget. Should long-term-care costs be only 10 percent more than most predictions, Medicare spending would increase by $5 billion. This argues for a cautious, gradual implementation of any new benefit to assure adequate control.

Second, if Medicare expands payment of long-term-institutional care, it moves away from a traditional medical orientation by reimbursing housing and maintenance costs. If Medicare is perceived to be financing the living expenses that prudent elders should have planned and saved for, the program may lose political support among young taxpayers. This concern could be addressed by having beneficiaries contribute a share of nursing home costs, a contribution that could be viewed as payment for the expenses of room and board (Bishop, 1981; Blumenthal et al., 1986).

Long-term-care benefits could be incorporated into the Medicare program in a variety of ways. Perhaps the most important issue of program design involves the choice between a voluntary and mandatory program. Making coverage a voluntary choice ensures that no beneficiary feels forced to pay premiums for long-term-care coverage, premiums that could be substantial even if subsidized through federal taxes.

Nevertheless, a voluntary public program is subject to the same problems of adverse selection as is private insurance. To avoid these problems, most proposals based on voluntary enrollment establish a cut-off age. Once beneficiaries pass this age—typically 70 years—they are no longer allowed to buy into the program (Auerbach, 1982; Davis and Rowland, 1986). Such an option may require too much foresight by elders. It also raises difficult questions about the responsibility of society to those who failed to purchase Medicare coverage of long-term care but later incur catastrophic expenses. It may only add another premium payment to an already fragmented set of coverages, exacerbating problems of complexity, cost shifting and fragmentation that are part of the current system.

Case Management Services

The elderly are confronted by a confusing array of health needs and services. The majority do not fully understand either what their insurance covers (Cafferata, 1984b) or what services are available (Holmes et al., 1983). Physicians often lack the necessary information or patience to successfully oversee elders' health care (U.S. General Accounting Office, 1981). As a result, beneficiaries may not receive care when needed (Branch and Nemeth, 1985).

The term *case management* has been used to refer to various types of remedial programs. Some would simply provide elders with information about their options for care, others would also assess elders' health needs and still others would make decisions on beneficiaries' behalf, directing them to certain services or acting as gatekeepers to restrict or control the use of services (Beatrice, 1981). Proposals for paying for case management through Medicare thus differ by whether they would inform, assess or make choices for beneficiaries (Cuccaro, 1980; Inspector General, 1981; Somers, 1982).

Proposals for Medicare-based case management also differ in two other respects. Some would place the physician in the role of the case manager; others would substitute an interdisciplinary team of professionals (Rowe, 1985). Some case-management systems would be limited to those elders at highest risk of institutionalization (Ruchlin et al., 1982); others would be made available to all beneficiaries (Breslow and Somers, 1977; Somers, 1982).

None of these various case management functions are being adequately provided under the current array of public and private coverages (Piktialis, 1986). Medicaid has been at the forefront in establishing various types of case-management programs (Hekman, 1984). As noted earlier, however, fragmentation of coverage among Medicare, Medicaid and Medigap plans makes coordination of care difficult (Cuccaro, 1980). Case management is further disrupted when elders lose and regain Medicaid eligibility as their income fluctuates.[10]

Medicare-based case management could overcome some of these limitations. Because Medicare covers a broad array of services and virtually the entire elder population, it could tie the power of the purse string to case-managers' decisions, greatly enhancing their efficacy. Because beneficiaries stay enrolled in Medicare, there is no disruption of case-management functions due to sporadic eligibility.

Concern for cost control has uncertain implications for the prospect of incorporating case management into Medicare. The cost of the case-management services themselves are reasonably predictable. These depend primarily on the number of functions case management includes: the more expansive the program, the more expensive the coverage. Based on the experience of existing small-scale programs, we estimate that costs of providing case management to all Medicare beneficiaries would range from $3 billion to $12 billion annually, the low figure corresponding to the provision of information only; the high figure including comprehensive assessment and monitoring of the health and health care of the elderly. These costs could be reduced by targeting the program to elders who are most at risk of institutionalization or high levels of service use (Schlesinger et al., 1984). Such targeting might limit annual costs to between $500 million and $2 billion (Harvard Medicare Project, 1986).

Less certain, however, is the indirect impact on use of other Medicare-covered services. Case managers may increase utilization by detecting unmet needs; conversely, they may reduce program costs by limiting inappropriate use of services (Lave, 1985). Experience with past and ongoing demonstration projects suggests that the more case management is targeted to high-risk elders, the more likely it is to reduce rather than increase costs (U.S. General Accounting Office, 1982c; Piktialis and MacAdam, 1984). Comprehensive programs appear to increase program costs on the order of 5 to 10 percent (Kemper, et al., 1986). Carefully targeted programs might reduce the costs of care for the target population by an equal percentage.

The political salience of case management is difficult to assess. Elders are becoming more concerned with obtaining reliable sources of information (Greenfield, 1986; Kerschner, 1986). On the other hand, many elders are probably sufficiently ill-informed that they do not even recognize their lack of information (Cafferata, 1984a). In addition, some elders resist the concept of gatekeepers who may limit their choice of acute care providers or services, though elders may be more accepting of case managment of long-term care (Friedman et. al., 1984).

Support may be more forthcoming from younger American who are increasingly enrolled in case-managed forms of private insurance. Most commercial insurers, for example, now require enrollees to obtain prior authorizations from the plan to use various types of services (Goldsmith, 1984). If case management were introduced to the Medicare program toward this same end, it would likely be favorably perceived as making Medicare as prudent a purchaser of health services as is the private sector.

Case-managment systems that provide information may strike the best balance of political support from beneficiaries and younger generations. Though such systems could not control costs or reduce inappropriate treatment to the same extent as more aggressive interventions, they also do not restrict elders' choices. They should thus be more popular among beneficiaries. Providing information can be justified to younger taxpayers as a means of making elders more astute consumers, thus reducing program costs and everyone's tax burden (Firman, 1985). Over time, as Americans become more familiar with insurance that requires prior authorization for care, more extensive case-management systems will likely become more politically acceptable.

The implementation of case management also depends in part on who is being asked to do the managing: physicians or a broader team of professionals. The academic literature presents a mixed assessment of the relative effectiveness of each approach (U.S. General Accounting Office, 1979; Rowe, 1985). On one hand, physicians already have regular contact with most beneficiaries and are familiar with their needs for medical care. On the other hand, doctors may have limited knowledge about the broader range of economic and social needs of the elderly or the availability of long-term care services in the community. In all likelihood, however, any case-management system would include a physican both for medical expertise and for the system to be politically viable (Schlesinger et al., 1984).

Social Services

Most of the 5 million chronically impaired older Americans require some help in their home to continue living in the community. About 20 percent of this help currently comes through home care agencies, the rest through the aid of family and friends (Manton and Liu, 1984; Doty, 1986). In the absence of this support elders are more likely to be institutionalized or to require other health care services (U.S. General Accounting Office, 1979; Arling and McAuley, 1983; Lave, 1985).

To prevent or delay institutionalization it has been suggested that Medicare broaden the array of services it reimburses beyond those narrowly defined as medical. These might include homemaker services (U.S. General Accounting Office, 1982c) or "respite care" (either in-home services or temporary stays in a nursing home or adult day-care unit) to relieve the stress on family caregivers (Doty, 1986).

Including nonmedical support services under Medicare coverage is likely to be supported by beneficiaries and the children of those who use the services. The elderly prefer independent living arrangements and wish to avoid burdening family and friends (Louis Harris, 1982). Family members who care for impaired elders prefer formal support services to any other type of assistance, including cash benefits (Doty, 1986).

Many of the benefits of these services, though, are psychological: they relieve stress on elders and their caretakers. To this point social services have not been shown to significantly and consistently reduce institutionalization or the use of other health care services (Weissert et al., 1980; U.S. General Accounting Office, 1982c; Doty, 1986).[11] Because the benefits produced by these services tend to be intangible, it may prove difficult to muster broader political support—beyond those who actually benefit from the service—to expand Medicare's budget to pay for them.

Extending Medicare coverage to social services also runs the risk of hard-to-control costs. Some fear that beneficiaries would apply for services even if they are not needed. Others see families abandoning their traditional roles as caregivers, leading to wholesale substitution of formal services (Doty, 1986). Costs of covering these services are hard to predict because the extent of this substitution is difficult to forecast.[12] Again, costs could be reduced and more readily controlled by targeting coverage to beneficiaries. Nonetheless, because small misestimates in the amount of substitution between informal and formal care could result in large differences in estimated cost (Pillemer, 1984), policymakers are likely to remain quite wary about coverage reforms of this type.

To control the potential for substitution of formal for informal care, social support services could be authorized only through a case manager. Alternatively, caps on program expenditures could be established for each enrollee—as with the hospice program—or for a group of beneficiaries in a prepaid health plan. Experiments are currently being conducted on the latter approach, termed a social/health maintenance organization or (S/HMO) (Diamond and Berman, 1981; Davis and Rowland, 1986). The S/HMOs have the potential to reduce costs and improve quality of care by creating incentives for substitution between health and social services.

Caution, however, seems in order. We as yet know little about the most appropriate ways to combine health and social services in a prepaid setting. Organizations given the responsibility to provide both types of care may still become overly medicalized, dominated by the interests of health care providers (Farrow et al., 1981). Moreover, because prepaid plans do not face the full societal costs of chronic illness, they may undersupply some needed services (Schlesinger, 1986) (see Chapter 7). These concerns suggest that the programs of integrating health and social services will not be resolved simply by placing them in a prepaid organization, and that more needs to be learned before S/HMOs can be seriously considered for widespread adoption.

Nor is it apparent that Medicare is the appropriate public progam to pay for support services. Although private insurers are unlikely to provide coverage, being strictly medically oriented (Meiners, 1983), state Medicaid programs have begun to incorporate nonmedical services under Section 2176, home and community-based waivers. These waivers, authorized by Congress in 1982, give states more discretion in determining eligibility so that services can be provided to any elder who would have become eligible if placed in a nursing home. As of 1985, there were 86 waivers granted to 46 states, though most of these have been used for local or regional demonstrations rather than statewide programs (Doty et al., 1985). Not only do states have growing experience in this area, they also control the allocation of Title XX funds, another major source of financing for social services. Therefore, coordination of funding streams may be more effective at the state level.

The most serious disadvantage to basing nonmedical programs under Medicaid is that, even with the waivers, eligibility is restricted to groups with more limited financial resources, though the problems of chronic illness are not limited to this group. This restriction may also make more difficult broader coordination of medical services (paid by Medicare) and social services (paid by Medicaid). In spite of these limitations, the historic ties of social services to state administration seem, on balance, to favor a state-based approach under a reformed Medicaid program.

Mental Health Care

Several recent studies have found that Medicare beneficiaries are not receiving adequate mental health care. Over 60 percent of the elderly with mental health care needs were not receiving treatment, more than for any other age group (Shapiro et al, 1985). Even if one takes into account differences in income, education and the perceived social stigma of mental illness, the elderly still use significantly fewer mental health care services (Leaf et al., 1985; Shapiro et al., 1985). "Those age 65 and over reported fewer mental health related contacts. . . . This suggests that older Americans may not be receiving the advantage of recent developments in the treatment of psychiatric disorders and the increased availability of mental health services" (Leaf et al., 1985, pp. 1333–34).

Proposals for expanding Medicare's coverage of mental health care adopt either of two approaches. The first calls for "coverage for mental health care services . . . on an equal basis with physical health care services" (Federal Council on Aging, 1978, p. 94). The second would expand Medicare benefits to make them equivalent to coverage available to the average working American (Harrington, 1982). Because Medicare's inpatient coverage is, by the standards of private insurance, fairly generous, this latter approach would have the greatest impact on outpatient coverage, raising the current $250 annual ceiling to between $1,500 and $2,000 a year.

By several of our criteria, extended mental health care coverage under Medicare seems both feasible and desirable. Despite common perceptions to the contrary, broad mental health care benefits do not lead to uncontrollable utilization. Private policies with relatively generous coverages have had histories of relatively stable use of psychiatric benefits (Sharfstein and Magnas, 1975; Krizay, 1982).

> Common myths about mental illness include notions about the ubiquity of such illness and the optional or even recreational nature of treatment. If everyone is sick and treatments are fun, then costs can go through the roof when someone else is paying the bill. But the evidence from empirical cost studies is exactly the opposite. . . . The issue then, is not one of breaking the bank, or uncontrollable costs" (Sharfstein et al., 1984, p. 29).

Extrapolating from this private experience, it seems likely that the costs of liberalized mental health care benefits under Medicare would be on the order of $1 billion to $2 billion annually.[13]

It is also not likely that Medicaid programs or private plans will adequately cover mental health care. Medicaid coverage of psychiatric care varies greatly from one state to another. Some programs impose ceilings as restrictive as those in Medicare. Forty percent of private Medigap plans offer no mental health coverage; others have, at best, very limited coverage (Cafferata, 1984b). Nor are most elders likely to voluntarily purchase more coverage in the future. Many are either unaware of their limited mental health care benefits or fear the social stigma of mental illness (Cafferata, 1984a; U.S. General Accounting Office, 1982b).

To what extent can Medicare coverage promote more adequate treatment of psychiatric illness? Though no change in the program will eliminate the perceived stigma of mental disorders, a well-publicized expansion of Medicare coverage might help legitimize treatment. In addition, expanded coverage will increase utilization, whatever the perceived stigma or other barriers to adequate care (McGuire, 1981). Thus, although it seems unlikely that Medicare coverage would in itself lead to adequate care and although it is difficult to predict exactly how much utilization would increase, it would undoubtedly be an improvement over the current coverage provisions.

Whether this improvement would be sufficiently pronounced to generate political support for the reform is another question. Although some politicians have called the current gaps in coverage (and the associated high rates of untreated mental illness) "a matter of the highest priority" and "a tragedy of enormous proportions" (Harrington, 1982, pp. 30–31), political support for mental health care financing has had a somewhat checkered past (Foley and Sharfstein, 1983). Moreover, the very stigmatization that discourages the elderly from purchasing private insurance coverage may also inhibit their lobbying to expand Medicare benefits for these services.[14]

Again, it may prove easier to generate support from younger taxpayers through an appeal to equity. Over the past decade a wave of state-legislated mandates have required that private insurance policies provide a minimum level of mental health care benefits. These minimum requirements, particularly for outpatient care, are often more generous than is Medicare's current coverage (Sharfstein et al., 1984). This suggests that broad-based political support may exist for liberalization of benefits, at least up to these minimum levels.

Preventive Services and Primary Care

Many elders see a physician regularly to be treated for chronic illness. Nonetheless, there are some beneficiaries who go for long periods without contact with a health care provider: Over 3 million elders have gone two or more years since seeing a physician (U.S. Department of Health and Human Services, 1984). A substantial number of elders fail to report symptoms of illness (Brody and Kleban, 1981). Seventeen percent of those over the age of 70 reported that they had not seen a physician in the previous year even though they felt unwell (Branch and Nemeth, 1985). Illnesses that go undiagnosed are likely to become more difficult and more costly to treat when they eventually are detected (Bonanno and Wetle, 1984).

To promote more timely diagnosis and treatment of illness it has been proposed that Medicare coverage foster more health promotion and disease prevention. This could involve educating elders on "symptom recognition, self-care, when to see the doctor, and similar matters" (Somers, 1984, p. 854) or providing reimbursement for specific diagnostic services or tests. Some plans would include this as a part of the standard Medicare coverage, others as an optional rider (Logsdon et al., 1984).

Although improved primary and preventive care is almost always favored in principle, it can be difficult to identify specific services for which Medicare coverage would be feasible and would improve the health of beneficiaries. Many forms of diagnostic testing and screening for the general population have been criticized as either ineffective or more costly than they are worth (Russell, 1986). For the elderly, health promotion through changes in behavior has also become controversial. Recent studies have produced conflicting evidence about the health benefits of reducing smoking, alcohol use and weight (Wingard et al., 1982; Branch and Jette, 1984; Jajich et al., 1984). Until these controversies are resolved, it may prove difficult to muster political support for a broadly defined goal of prevention.

It has been argued, though, that for the elderly the most important aspect of health promotion is the early detection and treatment of disease. This form of prevention may thus prove more productive for Medicare beneficiaries than for the general population (Besdine, 1982).

But Medicare may not be the most appropriate program for covering such preventive services. The costs of preventive care are not large, so that the major financial barriers owing to lack of coverage are felt primarily by the poor (Branch and Nemeth, 1985). Elders with limited incomes who are eligible for Medicaid have, in many states, fairly extensive coverage of primary care and diagnostic testing (Sawyer et al., 1983). Primary care for elders most affected by lack of coverage might therefore be improved most cost-effectively by requiring uniform national eligibility in the Medicaid program, not by changes in Medicare.

However, a substantial number of elders—between 1 and 2 million—do not see a physician when sick because of problems of transportation or inability to obtain an appointment (Branch and Nemeth, 1985). The primary care needs of this group may be best addressed through changes in Medicare coverage. By paying for outreach visits through home health agencies, the program could facilitate primary care for beneficiaries who might have difficulty gaining access to physician services. The costs of this coverage would neither be large nor difficult to predict or control. For example, if Medicare paid for a routine physical examination only for those beneficiaires who had not seen a provider in the previous year, coverage might cost as little as $500 million a year (Harvard Medicare project, 1986). Promoting more contact with health care providers could, of course, lead to additional treatment that could further increase Medicare spending. At the same time, early detection and treatment of illness will likely enhance the efficacy of treatment and to some extent reduce costs (Bonanno and Wetle, 1984). The net effect of these two outcomes is unclear, though there seems little potential for large increases in program spending. On balance then, covering home health screening visits for elders who had not recently seen a physician seems both desirable and feasible.

The Costs of Accumulated Small Expenses

A number of health care purchases are not individually expensive but can accumulate to become a substantial burden for the chronically ill elder. These include drugs, dental care and hearing and vision aids (Feder and Holahan, 1979). The average elder in the community requires 10 prescriptions a year; over 90 percent of the elderly need eyeglasses or contact lenses (Pegels, 1980; Waldo and Lazenby, 1984)

In the absence of insurance coverage, these needs often go unmet. Surveys indicate that a quarter of the elderly have such inadequate prescriptions that their glasses do not help and may, in fact, hinder their vision (Pegels, 1980). Similarly, "the dental needs of most elderly have been neglected . . . because dental insurance benefits usually end with retirement" (Neissen, 1984, p. 84).

The consequences of inadequate care can be serious. More than 10 percent of the elderly are legally blind as a result of untreated glaucoma and cataract conditions; inadequate dental care can impair the nutrition and thus the overall health of the elderly (Pegels, 1980). A recent study of elders' purchasing of prescription drugs found that when the elderly had to pay for these medicines, about one third of the time they failed to obtain drugs that clinicians judged vital to their health (Soumerai et al., 1986).

To improve elders access to these services it has been suggested that Medicare cover such costs. Because each individual purchase is not expensive, coverage might take the form of a stop-loss provision that pays for services only after a beneficiary has accumulated large annual expenditures.

These ancillary expenses meet several of our criteria for feasible coverage expansion. Cost control does not appear to be a problem. Several of these services—vision and hearing aids, dental care—will be used only a limited number of times by each beneficiary (Waldo and Lazenby, 1984). The costs of other services, such as prescription drugs, could be limited by introducing coverage as a stop-loss provision. If, for example, Medicare paid only the drug costs for the 5 percent of beneficiaries with the largest expenses for medicines, costs of coverage would be about $1.5 billion annually, a fifth of elders' total spending on prescription drugs (Feder and Holahan, 1979).

Coverage of these expenses would also gain the political support of many elders. Surveys conducted by the AARP show that beneficiaries, particularly those with limited incomes, favored coverage of ancillary costs.

Coverage would, however, also face several challenges. It is unclear whether younger taxpayers would be willing to pay for services that are not included in a majority of their own policies. It is also unclear that Medicare has any real advantage in providing these coverages. Elders with adequate resources should increasingly be able to purchase coverage through private supplementary plans—as dental coverage, for example, becomes more common in employer group plans, commercial insurers will more readily offer it as an option in Medigap plans.

Because these costs are most problematic for elders with limited incomes, they are perhaps best addressed by reform of the Medicaid program. Many Medicaid programs already cover costs for prescription drugs and eyeglasses for those who are Medicaid eligible (Sawyer et al., 1983). Other states have instituted programs to pay the costs of prescription drugs for elders with limited incomes, but who are not enrolled in Medicaid. More comprehensive coverage could be provided by mandating more uniform state-based programs; arguably, these better focus coverage on elders most in need.

The Potential for Medicare Service Coverage Reform

Medicare coverage of health services has changed little over the past two decades. This stasis was produced, ironically, as much through efforts of the program's supporters as by its detractors. Increased reform, however, appears possible in the near future. As elders become more aware of the program's current limitations, they will more readily support broad-based reform. As society as a whole becomes more conscious of the problems of an aging population, there will be increased support for programs addressing the needs of the chronically ill. As the shortcomings of Medicaid become more widely appreciated, Americans will undoubtedly seek other means of paying for the long-term care needed by themselves and their parents. As we become more experienced with different models of case management and utilization review, we will be better able to cover services for the chronically ill without losing control of program spending.

Virtually all the proposals considered in this chapter have merit because they address important unmet needs of the elderly. However, we have argued that not all are equally feasible politically, fiscally or administratively. Some of these problems may be better addressed by programs other than Medicare. Others would be feasible and effective under Medicare only if targeted to particular groups of beneficiaries or limited to certain services.

In assessing the potential of these half-dozen types of services reform, we have tried to be foresighted, to consider how feasibility will be affected by what we are likely to learn over the next few years. Nonetheless, some of our thinking has been inevitably shaped by more short-term considerations. As a result, some reforms that seem infeasible today may prove manageable in another 5 or 10 years.

Views of the Medicare program change slowly. The program was initially conceived as a medical program, with reimbursable services defined largely in terms of those provided by physicians. It is increasingly recognized by geriatricians that health care for the elderly is not appropriately limited to medical care. Nonetheless, broad public perceptions of what is appropriate for Medicare coverage have not kept pace with this professional consensus. To the extent that these broader perceptions change in the future, it may become more feasible to incorporate coverage of social support services into Medicare.

Future improvements in our ability to control costs will make other services more feasible as well. At present, we know too little to definitively determine the effectiveness of using case management to target services to beneficiaries most in need or how best to structure case-management programs. As our experience with preadmission screening under Medicaid and utilization review in private insurance plans grows, Medicare will be able to make use of this knowledge and provide more comprehensive cost-effective coverage of services.

Perhaps the most important lesson from Medicare's first twenty-three years is identifying the fallacy of assuming that any program, however well conceived, will be able to meet the changing needs of its beneficiaries without itself changing. Not only must a program be designed to be flexible, but the program's proponents must also be willing to accept and to actively work for change. Attempts to preserve Medicare by freezing it in its original image will in the end only weaken it, leaving it unable to meet the goals for which it was initially designed.

NOTES

1. In 1972, Medicare coverage was extended to pay for the treatment of end-stage renal disease (ESRD). This was not, however, a program intended exclusively or even primarily for the elderly: only one quarter of all patients receiving dialysis are over the age of 65 (Eggars et al., 1984).

2. Nor can the elderly rely, as many of us do, on the advice of a physician in selecting health services. Most physicians know relatively little about the availability of long-term care services (U.S. General Accounting Office, 1981). Their knowledge of home health care and related services is particularly poor, leading them to unnecessarily direct their elder patients into nursing homes (U.S. General Accounting Office, 1979).

3. Regulations designed to protect elders from fraudulent practices also make it more difficult to introduce innovative new policies, thus reducing the flexibility that this mixed system of coverages was intended to provide (Meiners, 1983).

4. One survey found that between 30 and 50 percent of those who are initially admitted to a nursing home as private-pay patients convert to Medicaid coverage within a year (U.S. General Accounting Office, 1979).

5. This occurs most commonly in nursing homes when administrators pressure residents who have spent down to Medicaid eligibility to transfer to another facility (Pegels, 1980). This practice is illegal in most states. The same end can be achieved, however, by transferring Medicaid-eligible residents to a hospital for medical care. While hospitalized, their bed is then given to private-pay patients.

6. Most such patients require renal dialysis two to three times a week for the rest of their lives.

7. Pressure from the Office of Management and Budget did, though, dramatically reduce hospice reimbursement. This has inhibited the growth of the program, suggesting that its political support was not as strong as that for other parts of the program (Fraser, 1985).

8. Some proposals would extend Medicare coverage to only one of these services (U.S. Congressional Budget Office, 1977). Most reformers argue, however, that both services must be covered to insure that care is appropriately matched to beneficiaries' needs and that opportunities for cost-saving substitution are exploited.

9. "Actuaries fear that private insurers' liability cannot be limited adequately because of difficulties defining objectively this type of insurable event" (Brecher and Knickman, 1985, p. 249). Given the great conservatism shown by insurance companies in the development of long-term care, innovative expansions of coverage to home care seem unlikely (Jazweicki, 1986).

10. Several states have established informational systems for elders, but these have had very limited budgets and rely largely on volunteers. It seems unrealistic to rely entirely on voluntarism to meet the needs of all beneficiaries, unless the program is supported by some broader institutional framework.

11. As with case management, the key issue seems to be one of targeting. Support services may reduce institutionalization for high-risk groups, but this effect is diluted and difficult to measure because many low-risk elders also use services (U.S. General Accounting Office, 1982c).

12. We estimate that a broad coverage of homemaker services could cost as much as $20 billion a year; respite care $2 billion to $3 billion.

13. We assume, in this estimate, that care of Alzheimer's disease would be covered under long-term care, not mental health provisions.

14. There is a growing popular recognition of the problems of Alzheimer's disease among the elderly. This may stimulate support for more general interventions for dealing with the mental health care needs of this population (Piktialis, 1986).

REFERENCES

Arling, G., and W. J. McAuley. 1983. The Feasibility of Public Payments for Family Caregiving. *Gerontologist* 23:300–306.

Auerbach, A. 1982. Medicare Plan C: A Long-Term Care Proposal. *Generations* 7 (Spring):48–53.

Bayer, R., and D. Callahan. 1985. Medicare Reform: Social and Ethical Perspectives. *Journal of Health Politics, Policy and Law* 10 (3):533–47.

Beatrice, D. F. 1981. Case Management: A Policy for Long-Term Care. In *Reforming the Long-Term Care System*, ed. J. J. Callahan, Jr., and S. S. Wallack, pp. 121–61. Lexington, MA: D. C. Heath.

Besdine, R. W. 1982. Database of Geriatric Medicine. In *Health and Disease in Old Age*, ed. J. W. Rowe and R. W. Besdine. Boston: Little, Brown.

Binstock, R. H. 1985. The Oldest Old: A Fresh Perspective or Compassionate Ageism Revisited. *Milbank Memorial Fund Quarterly* 63 (2):420–51.

Bishop, C. E. 1981. A Compulsory National Long-Term Care Insurance Program. In *Reforming the Long-Term Care System*, ed. J. J. Callahan, Jr., and S. S. Wallack, pp. 61–93. Lexington, MA: D. C. Heath.

Blumenthal, David, Mark Schlesinger, Pamela Brown Drumheller et al. 1986. The Future of Medicare. *New England Journal of Medicine* 314 (11):722–28.

Bonanno, J. B., and T. Wetle. 1984. HMO Enrollment of Medicare Recipients: An Analysis of Incentives and Barriers. *Journal of Health Politics, Policy and Law* 9 (1):41–62.

Branch, L., and A. Jette. 1984. Personal Health Practice and Mortality Among the Elderly. *American Journal of Epidemiology* 116:765–75.

Branch, L. G., and K. T. Nemeth. 1985. When Elders Fail to Visit Physicians. *Medical Care* 23 (11):1265–76.

Brecher, C., and J. Knickman. 1985. A Reconsideration of Long-Term Care Policy. *Journal of Health Politics, Policy and Law* 10 (2):245–73.

Breslow, L., and A. Somers. 1977. The Lifetime Health-Monitoring Program: A Practical Approach to Preventive Medicine. *New England Journal of Medicine* 296 (9):601–8.

Brody, E. M., and M. H. Kleban. 1981. Physical and Mental Health Symptoms of Older People: Who Do They Tell? *Journal of the American Geriatrics Society* 29:442–49.

Butler, L. H., and P. W. Newacheck. 1981. Health and Social Factors Relevant to Long Term Care Policy. In *Policy Options in Long-Term Care*, ed. J. Meltzer, F. Farrow and H. Richman, pp. 38–77. Chicago: University of Chicago Press.

Cafferata, G. 1984a. *Knowledge of Their Health Insurance Coverage by the Elderly*. U.S. Department of Health and Human Services, Public Health Service, Office of the Assistant Secretary for Health, National Center for Health Services Research.

———. 1984b. *Private Health Insurance Coverage of the Medicare Population: Data Preview 18*. U.S. Department of Health and Human Services, Public Health Service, Office of the Assistant Secretary for Health, National Center for Health Services Research.

Callahan, J. J., Jr. 1981. Single Agency Option for Long-Term Care. In *Reforming the Long-Term Care System*, ed. J. J. Callahan, Jr., and S. S. Wallack, pp. 163–84. Lexington, MA: D. C. Heath.

Cuccaro, R. 1980. Testimony before the Committee on Labor and Human Resources and the Special Committee on Aging. U.S. Congress, Senate, 96th Congress, 2d session. Joint Hearing, November 23.

Davidson, S. M., and T. R. Marmor. 1980. *The Cost of Living Longer: National Health Insurance and the Elderly*. Lexington, MA: D. C. Heath.

Davis, K., and D. Rowland. 1986. *Medicare Policy: New Directions for Health and Long-Term Care*. Baltimore: Johns Hopkins University Press.

Diamond, L. M., and D. E. Berman. 1981. The Social/Health Maintenance Organization: A Single-Entry, Prepaid, Long-Term Care Delivery System. In *Reforming the Long-Term Care System*, ed. J. J. Callahan, Jr., and S. S. Wallack, pp. 185–213. Lexington, MA: Lexington Books.

Doty, P. 1986. Family Care of the Elderly: The Role of Public Policy. *Milbank Memorial Fund Quarterly* 64 (1):34–75.

Doty, P., K. Liu and J. Wiener. 1985. An Overview of Long-Term Care. *Health Care Financing Review* 6 (3):69–78.

Dunlop, B. 1983. The Medicare Hospice Benefit: Unanticipated Cost and Access Impacts? *Health Affairs* 2 (3):127–31.

Eggars, P. W., R. Connerton and M. McMullan. 1984. The Medicare Experience with End-Stage Renal Disease: Trends in Incidence, Prevalence, and Survival. *Health Care Financing Review* 5 (3):69–88.

Farrow, F., T. Joe, J. Meltzer et al. 1981. The Framework and Directions for Change. In *Policy Options in Long-Term Care*, ed. J. Meltzer, F. Farrow and H. Richman, pp. 1–37. Chicago: University of Chicago Press.

Feder, J. M. 1977. *Medicare: The Politics of Federal Hospital Insurance*. Lexington, MA: Lexington Books.

Feder, J., and J. Holahan. 1979. *Financing Health Care for the Elderly: Medicare, Medicaid, and Private Health Insurance*. Washington: Urban Institute Press.

Feder, J., and W. Scanlon. 1982. The Underused Benefit: Medicare's Coverage of Nursing Home Care. *Milbank Memorial Fund Quarterly* 60 (4):604–32.

Federal Council on Aging. 1978. *Public Policy and the Frail Elderly*. DHEW Publication No. (OHDS) 79-20959. Washington, DC.

Firman, J. 1985. Health Care Cooperatives: Innovations for Older People. *Health Affairs* 4(4):50–61.

Foley, H. A., and S. S. Sharfstein. 1983. *Madness and Government: Who Cares for the Mentally Ill?* Washington: American Psychiatric Press.

Fraser, I. 1985. Medicare Reimbursement for Hospice Care: Ethical and Policy Implications of Cost-Containment Strategies. *Journal of Health Politics, Policy and Law* 10 (3):565–78.

Friedman, B., S. A. LaTour and E. F. X. Hughes. 1984. A Medicare Voucher System: What Can It Offer? *Proceedings of the Conference on the Future of Medicare* Subcommittee on Health, Committee on Ways and Means, U.S. House of Representatives, 55–78.

Ginsburg, P. B. 1983. Market-Oriented Options in Medicare and Medicaid. In *Market Reforms in Health Care: Current Issues, New Directions, Strategic Decisions*, ed. J. A. Meyer, pp. 103–17. Washington: American Enterprise Institute for Public Policy Research.

Glenn, K. and T. Brazda, 1985. Medicaid Spending Slows Down. *Washington Report on Medicine and Health.* May 20.

Goldsmith, J. 1984. Death of a Paradigm: The Challenge to Competition. *Health Affairs* 3 (3):5–29.

Greenfield, C. A. 1986. Improving Elderly Access to Health Care Information. *Business and Health* 3 (7):26–30.

Gruenberg, L., and T. Willemain. 1982. Hospital Discharge Queues in Massachusetts. *Medical Care* 20 (2):188–98.

Hagen, R. 1986. Medigap Insurance: Pitfalls and Progress. *Business and Health* 3 (5):25–30.

Harrington, G. 1982. *The Medicare Answer Book.* New York: Harper and Rowe.

Hartke, V. 118 *Congressional Record* 33003 (1972).

Harvard Medicare Project. 1986. *Medicare: Coming of Age. A Proposal for Reform.* Boston: Division of Health Policy Research and Education, Harvard University.

Health Insurance Association of America. 1983. *Source Book of Health Insurance Data 1982–1983.* Washington: Author.

Hekman, E. 1984. *States' Efforts at Health Care Cost Containment.* National Conference of States' Legislatures. Denver, CO.

Holmes, D., J. Teresi and M. Holmes. 1983. Differences Among Black, Hispanic and White People in Knowledge About Long-Term Care Services. *Health Care Financing Review* 5 (2):51–65.

Iglehart, J. K. 1985. Medicare Turns to HMOs. *New England Journal of Medicine* 312 (2):132–37.

Inspector General. U.S. Department of Health and Human Services. 1981. *Service Delivery Assessment on Long-Term Care.*

Jajich, C., A. Ostfield and D. Freeman. 1984. Smoking and Coronary Heart Disease Mortality in the Elderly. *Journal of the American Medical Association* 252:2831–34.

Jazwiecki, T. 1986. Financing Options for Long-Term Care Services. *Business and Health* 3 (3):18–24.

Kane, R. A., and R. L. Kane. 1985. The Feasibility of Universal Long-Term Care Benefits. *New England Journal of Medicine* 312 (21):1357–64.

Kemper, P., R. Brown, G. Carcagno, et al. 1986. *The Evaluation of the National Long-Term Care Demonstration: Final Report.* Princeton: Mathematical Policy Research.

Kerschner, P. A. 1986. Are DRGs Affecting Just the Elderly? *Business and Health* 3 (5):31–37.

Krizay, J. 1982. Federal Employees' Experience as a Guide to the Cost of Insuring Psychiatric Services in the Various States. *American Journal of Psychiatry* 139:866–871.

Lambert, Z. V. 1980. Elderly Consumers' Knowledge Related to Medigap Protection Needs. *Journal of Consumer Affairs.* 2:434.

Lave, J. R. 1985. Cost Containment Policies in Long-Term Care. *Inquiry* 22 (1):7–23.

Leaf, P. J., M. M. Livingston, G. L. Tischler et al. 1985. Contact with Health Professionals for the Treatment of Psychiatric and Emotional Problems. *Medical Care* 23 (12):1322–37.

Levit, K. R., H. Lazenby, D. R. Waldo et al. 1985. National Health Expenditures, 1984. *Health Care Financing Review* 7 (1):1–35.

Logsdon, D. N., M. A. Rosen and S. G. Karson. 1984. Health Insurance for Preventive Services. *Journal of Insurance and Medicine* 15 (1):2–9.

Louis Harris and Associates, Inc. 1982. *Priorities and Expectations for Health and Living Circumstances: A Survey of the Elderly in Five English-Speaking Countries*. A Study for the Commonwealth Fund. New York.

Lowrie, E. G., and C. L. Hampers. 1982. Proprietary Dialysis and the End-Stage Renal Disease Program. *Dialysis & Transplantation* 11 (3):191–204.

Manton, K., and K. Liu. 1984. *The Future Growth of the Long-Term Care Population: Projections Based on the 1977 National Nursing Home Survey and the 1982 Long-Term Care Survey*. Paper presented at the Third National Leadership Conference on Long-Term Care Issues, Washington, March 7–9.

Marmor, T. R. 1969. The Congress: Medicare Politics and Policy. In *American Political Institutions and Public Policy: Five Contemporary Studies*, ed. A. P. Sindler, pp. 3–66. Boston: Little, Brown.

Marmor, Theodore R. 1970. *The Politics of Medicare*. Chicago: Aldine.

McGuire, T. G. 1981. *Financing Psychotherapy: Costs, Effects, and Public Policy*. Cambridge, MA: Ballinger.

Meiners, M. 1983. The Case for Long-Term Care Insurance. *Health Affairs* 2 (2):55–79.

———. 1984. *The State of the Art in Long-Term Care Insurance*. Paper prepared for the Health Care Financing Administration Conference on Long-Term Care Financing and Delivery Systems: Exploring Some Alternatives, January 24.

Meyer, J. 1983. Introduction. In *Market Reforms in Health Care: Current Issues, New Directions, Strategic Decisions*, ed. J. A. Meyer, pp. 1–11. Washington: American Enterprise Institute for Public Policy Research.

Monier, C., M. Makowiecki and M. Yessian. 1981. *Medicare Home Health Services: Policy Recommendations and Implications*. Office of Service Delivery Assessment, Office of the Inspector General, U.S. Department of Health and Human Services.

Morris, R., and P. Youket. 1981. The Long-Term Care Issues: Identifying the Problems and Potential Solutions. In *Reforming the Long-Term Care System*, ed. J. J. Callahan, Jr., and S. S. Wallack, pp. 11–28. Lexington, MA: D. C. Heath.

Muszynski, S., J. Brady and S. S. Sharfstein. 1983. *Coverage for Mental and Nervous Disorders: Summary of 300 Private Sector Health Insurance Plans*. Washington: American Psychiatric Press.

National Association for Home Care. 1986. *The Attempted Dismantling of the Medicare Home Health Benefit*. A report to Congress. Washington, DC.

Neissen, L. 1984. Extending Dental Insurance Through Retirement. *Special Care in Dentistry* March–April.

New York Times. 1986. Nursing Costs Force Elderly to Sue Spouses. March 6:1.

Pauly, M. Taxation, Health Insurance and Market Failure in the Medical Economy. *Journal of Economic Literature* 24 (2):629–675.

Pegels, C. C. 1980. *Health Care and the Elderly*. Rockville, MD: Aspen Systems Corporation.

Piktialis, D. 1986. Private Long-Term Care Insurance: A Partial Solution? *American Journal of Alzheimer's Care and Related Disorders* 1 (1):37–43.

Piktialis, D., and M. A. MacAdam. 1984. Experiments and Demonstration in Shaping and Coordination. In *Older Veterans: Linking VA and Community Resources*, ed. T. Wetle and J. W. Rowe, 93–157. Cambridge: Harvard University Press.

Pillemer, K. 1984. How Do We Know How Much We Need? Problems in Determining Need for Long-Term Care. *Journal of Health Politics, Policy and Law* 9 (2):281–90.

Rosenfeld, A. 1982. *Home Health Services and Long-Term Care: A Two-State Comparison*. Discussion Paper. University Health Policy Consortium, Brandeis University, Waltham, MA.

Rosenwaike, I. 1985. A Demographic Portrait of the Oldest Old. *Milbank Memorial Fund Quarterly* 63 (2):187–205.

Rowe, J. W. 1985. Health Care of the Elderly. *New England Journal of Medicine* 312 (13):827–35.

Ruchlin, H. S., J. N. Morris and G. M. Eggert. 1982. Management and Financing of Long-Term Care Services: A New Approach to a Chronic Problem. *New England Journal of Medicine* 306 (2):101–5.

Russell, L. B. 1986. *Is Prevention Better Than Cure?* Washington: Brookings Institution.

Sawyer, D., M. Ruther, A. Pagan-Berlucchi et al. 1983. *The Medicare and Medicaid Data Book, 1983*. U.S. Department of Health and Human Services, Health Care Financing Administration, Office of Research and Demonstrations. HCFA Pub. No. 03156.

Schlesinger, M. 1986. On the Limits of Expanding Health Care Reform: Chronic Care in Prepaid Settings. *Milbank Quarterly* 64 (2):189–215.

Schlesinger, M., T. Wetle and J. H. Morse. 1984. Improving Care of the Older Veteran: Issues and Options. In *Older Veterans: Linking VA and Community Resources*, ed. T. Wetle and J. W. Rowe, 409–33. Cambridge: Harvard University Press.

Shapiro, S., E. A. Skinner, M. Kramer et al. 1985. Measuring Need for Mental Health Services in a General Population. *Medical Care* 23 (9):1033–43.

Sharfstein, S. S., and H. L. Magnas. 1975. Insuring Intensive Psychotherapy. *American Journal of Psychiatry* 132:1252–56.

Sharfstein, S. S., S. Muszynski and E. Myers. 1984. *Health Insurance and Psychiatric Care: Update and Appraisal.* Washington: American Psychiatric Press.

Sokoloff, S., and W. Sota. 1985. *Private Long-Term Care Insurance: View of the Nation and the Commonwealth.* Paper presented for the Public Policy Committee, Massachusetts Gerontology Association, September.

Soldo, B. J., and K. G. Manton 1985. Changes in the Health Status and Service Needs of the Oldest Old: Current Patterns and Future Trends. *Milbank Memorial Fund Quarterly* 63 (2):286–323.

Somers, A. 1982. Long-Term Care For the Elderly and Disabled. *New England Journal of Medicine* 307 (4):221–26.

———. 1984. Why Not Try Preventing Illness as a Way of Controlling Medicare Costs? *New England Journal of Medicine* 311 (13):853–56.

Soumerai, S., J. Avorn, D. Ross-Degnan and S. Gortmaker. 1987. Payment Restrictions for Prescription Drugs Under Medicaid. *New England Journal of Medicine* 317 (9):550–556.

Thompson, Frank J. 1981. *Health Policy and the Bureaucracy: Politics and Implementation.* Cambridge: MIT Press.

Torrey, B. B. 1985. Sharing Increasing Costs on Declining Income: The Visible Dilemma of the Invisible Aged. *Milbank Memorial Fund Quarterly* 63 (2):377–394.

U.S. Congress. House. Select Committee on Aging. 1985. *Twentieth Anniversary of Medicare and Medicaid: Americans Still at Risk.* 99th Congress, 1st session. Hearing.

U.S. Congress. Senate. Committee on Finance. 1970. *Medicare and Medicaid: Problems, Issues, and Alternatives.* 91st Congress, 1st session.

U.S. Congressional Budget Office. 1977. *Long-Term Care for the Elderly and Disabled.*

U.S. Department of Health and Human Services, National Center for Health Statistics, Public Health Service. 1984. *Health, United States 1984.* DHHS Pub. No. (PHS) 85–1232.

U.S. General Accounting Office. 1979. *Entering a Nursing Home: Costly Implications for Medicaid and the Elderly.* Pub. No. PAD–80–12.

———. 1981. *Medicare Home Health Services: A Difficult Program to Control.* Pub. No. HRD–81–155.

———. 1982a. *Assessment of the Use of Tax Credits for Families Who Provide Health Care to Disabled Elderly Relatives.* Pub. No. GAO/IPE–82–7.

———. 1982b. *The Elderly Remain in Need of Mental Health Services*. Pub. No. GAO/HRD–82–112.

———. 1982c. *The Elderly Should Benefit from Expanded Home Health Care but Increasing These Services Will Not Ensure Cost Reductions*. Pub. No. GAO/IPE–83–1.

Vladeck, B. 1980. *Unloving Care: The Nursing Home Tragedy*. New York: Basic Books.

Waldo, D. R., and H. C. Lazenby. 1984. Demographic Characteristics and Health Care Use and Expenditures by the Aged in the United States: 1977–1984. *Health Care Financing Review* 69 (1):1–29.

Weissert, W. G. 1985. Estimating the Long-Term Care Population: Prevalence Rates and Selected Charactertistics. *Health Care Financing Review* 6 (4):83–91.

Weissert, W. G., T. H. Wan and B. B. Livieratos. 1980. *Effects and Costs of Day Care and Homemaker Services for the Chronically Ill: A Randomized Experiment*. DHEW Pub. No. (PHS) 79–3258.

Wingard, D., L. Berkman and R. Brand. 1982. A Multivariate Analysis of Health-Related Practices. *American Journal of Epidemiology* 116:765–75.

Winn, S., and K. McCaffree. 1979. Issues Involved in the Development of a Prepaid Capitation Plan for Long-Term Care Services. *Gerontologist* 19:184–90.

5

Medicare's Payment of Hospitals

JUDITH BENTKOVER
PHILIP CAPER
MARK SCHLESINGER
JOEL SULDAN

Every reimbursement system involves a clash of values. If payments are "generous," then beneficiaries will be freely admitted to health care facilities and treated with the full range of procedures deemed appropriate by health care professionals. These are worthy outcomes. Yet each has a flip side that is less attractive. Reimbursement systems that promote access may also encourage unnecessary use of medical care. Payment systems that encourage a full range of treatment in addition may lead to waste, inefficiency and excessive utilitization that can actually impair beneficiaries' health.

If we had the understanding to separate needed from unnecessary utilization or better treatment from wasteful excess, this knowledge could be built into the reimbursement system. Because we do not, payment methods that encourage some desirable goals work against others. To design reimbursement systems one must face trade-offs among desired outcomes.

When choosing how to pay providers, therefore, it is not simply a matter of identifying the "right" or "wrong" methods of reimbursement. Compromises must be made, and the best way to do this depends on how society values access to care relative to efficiency or quality of care. The history of Medicare's hospital reimbursement reflects a shift in these values. In the 1960s, hospital reimbursement was designed almost exclusively to encourage access to, and utilization of, services for beneficiaries. Rising hospital expenditures over the next two-plus decades, however, increased concern with cost control. This was embodied in Medicare's shift from cost-based retrospective reimbursement to prospective payment for hospital care. The transition has raised additional issues about how fairly Medicare's system of hospital payment now treats beneficiaries and providers.

Society's priorities are likely to change in the future just as they have in the past. It seems unlikely, however, that Medicare will at any time in the foreseeable future return to a system that pays hospitals as if price were no object. The principal challenge for policymakers is, thus, to design a reimbursement system that provides incentives for efficient delivery of care while preserving adequate levels of accessibility, quality and equity. A variety of alternative approaches have been proposed to do this, though not all are likely to prove equally workable.

The historical evolution of Medicare's hospital reimbursement and the options for future reform are examined later in this chapter. We assess the cost, complexity and potential efficacy of each proposed change. Whether these reforms eventually become a part of the Medicare program, though, depends largely on how Americans in the future choose to balance the conflicting values inherent in every reimbursement system. Factors influencing this choice are discussed throughout the chapter and summarized at its end.

On the Road to PPS and DRGs*

Medicare in the 1960s

To understand the history of hospital payment under Medicare it is useful to briefly review the development of the private insurance plans that came before it. Hospital reimbursement by insurers had its origin in the Blue Cross plans created across the country during the 1930s (Law, 1974).

Beginning with the first Blue Cross plan, organized in Texas at the height of the Depression, hospitals were paid on the basis of their costs. This proved generous to hospitals because it put them at no financial risk. It also encouraged a price-is-no-object philosophy, promoting more and greater use of technologies that increased both cost and quality of care. The incentives created by the payment system were no accident. The Blue Cross plans were established and, for most of their history, controlled by hospital associations (Feldstein, 1978). Consequently, the goals they favored were those of the administrators who ran the hospitals as well as the affiliated medical staff (Starr, 1982).

As Blue Cross plans spread across the United States in the 1930s and 1940s so did cost-based hospital reimbursement. As commercial insurance companies entered the hospital insurance field in the late 1940s and early 1950s, many adopted a system of charge-based payment that proved even more generous to hospitals.

During the post-World War II period, the spread of Blue Cross and commercial health insurance plans was given a boost by the burgeoning labor union movement and the widespread adoption of hospital insurance as a fringe benefit of employment. Growth was also favored by federal tax law that, in effect, subsidized the purchase of private insurance by excluding insurance benefits from taxable income (Pauly, 1986). Cost- and charge-based retrospective reimbursement of hospitals thus became part of the mainstream of American medicine.

When Medicare was adopted in 1965, provisions for paying hospitals were patterned after methods used by private insurers. This was done for several reasons. First, to win the support of the private insurance industry, Medicare's proponents agreed to use Blue Cross plans and commercial insurance companies as fiscal intermediaries (Thompson, 1981). It was thus natural to borrow their methods of paying hospitals. Second, at the time the legislation was written, there was some

*PPS—prospective payment system; DRGs—diagnosis-related groups.

concern that providers might boycott Medicare enrollees (Feder, 1977). It was, therefore, deemed wise to pay providers generously to encourage participation.

Third, Medicare was passed at the end of two decades of federal policy-making intended to promote greater access to higher-quality health services. In the quest for expanded health care resources, the federal Hill-Burton program had greatly increased the number of hospital beds (Lave and Lave, 1974). State and federal educational subsidies had increased the number of health professionals available to provide services in hospitals. A plethora of government research subsidies supported the development of the hospital-based medical technologies. Following in this tradition, it is not surprising that Medicare adopted a system of paying hospitals designed to promote these same goals.

Finally, the enactment of Medicare and Medicaid represented more than simply the provision of health insurance to the poor and the elderly. It embodied a commitment to provide these groups with access to the "mainstream" health care system. This required that Medicare reflect the goals of the rest of American medical care in the 1960s: that cost was no object and that the purpose of a reimbursement system was to promote high-quality care for all beneficiaries.

Medicare's provisions for hospital reimbursement worked in the following way. Each hospital nominated a fiscal intermediary to do its claims processing. The intermediary computed the hospitals's reasonable costs in accordance with a formula that took into account patient-care costs incurred, as well as other costs such as those related to capital. Care of each patient was reimbursed based on these allowable costs.

Medicare's system of hospital payment was, in fact, quite successful at promoting access to, and utilization of, hospital services (Feder, 1977; Davis and Schoen, 1978). This "success," though, led to new problems and the gradual evolution of new policy objectives over the next 10 years.

The 1970s: Cost Consciousness and Regulation

As early as 1970, the Senate Finance Committee was calling attention to Medicare's burgeoning budget. As yet, however, there was not great interest in changing the way in which Medicare paid hospitals. Instead, attempts were made to fine-tune the system through a series of regulatory initiatives that preserved the basic incentives of the reimbursement system.

Over the next several years, a series of reforms were incorporated into the Medicare program. The 1972 Social Security amendments authorized the establishment of price controls in the form of reimbursement limits for routine (room and board) costs (Section 223 limits). Also enacted in these amendments were the Professional Standards Review Organization (PSRO) program and provisions that authorized voluntary planning arrangements between state and federal governments (Section 1122 agreements).

The PSRO program established a national network of physician-operated, peer review agencies to monitor the quality and quantity of hospital services provided to Medicare beneficiaries. The intent of these reviews was to identify and discourage inappropriate use of hospital services.

Section 1122 agreements authorized the federal government to withhold reimbursement for treatment provided by new facilities not approved by the appropriate state-planning agency. The National Health Planning and Resource Development Act of 1974 required that certificate-of-need (CON) programs be established in all states to regulate the construction of health care facilities.

These regulatory controls proved insufficient to effectively counter the inflationary characteristics of Medicare's hospital reimbursement. Spending on hospital care continued to climb rapidly. Controls on routine hospital costs left ancillary services unregulated, and the prices for these nonroutine costs rose particularly quickly throughout the decade.

The impact of the PSRO program is unclear despite several studies that have examined the program's effect on hospitalization, procedure rates and costs of hospital care. Several of these studies indicate that peer review can have a beneficial impact and that procedure rates as well as patient days were decreased by PSRO activities (Mitchell et al., 1975; Lave and Leinhardt, 1976; Gertman et al., 1978). However, other studies conclude that PSROs have had no impact on hospital utilization (Bonner, 1976; Brook and Williams, 1976; Roemer, 1976; Dobson et al., 1978). According to the Congressional Budget Office (CBO), the PSRO progam operated at a net loss of between $0.30 and $0.60 for every dollar spent (U.S. Congressional Budget Office, 1980).[1]

Evaluations of CON programs have also offered mixed reviews. During the 1960s and 1970s, several researchers concluded that hospital utilization—and, therefore, expenditures—was positively related to the supply of available hospital beds (Roemer, 1961; Cheswick, 1974; May, 1975; Newhouse and Phelps, 1976). Those findings supported the notion that regional planning to reduce or control spending on new hospital facilities had the potential to significantly lower hospital costs. However, many subsequent studies have concluded that programs designed to regulate hospital construction had had, in practice, limited impact (Macro Systems, 1975; Hellinger, 1976; Rothenberg, 1976; Sloan and Steinwald, 1980; Policy Analysis/Urban Systems, 1981). "All the empirical evidence to date supports the conclusion that the massive certificate-of-need apparatus has had little effect on hospital expenditures" (Jaskow, 1981, p. 168).

Still more recent research, based on the analysis of data from several years, supports the theory that controls on facility construction can, with time, attain some cost savings. In particular, one study concluded that capital-investment behavior imposed by restrictive regulation is likely to show lagged rather than immediate effects (Howell, 1981). Other research has established that capital investment does provide an important impetus to the growth of total hospital expenditures. In particular, it was found that, on average, a dollar invested in hospital capital increased operating costs $0.22 (Bentkover et al., 1984).

Nonetheless, there is widespread agreement that CON programs are inadequate in themselves to control increases in hospital costs. Much the same can be said for all these regulatory controls taken together; at most, they only slightly slowed skyrocketing payments. Between 1967 and 1975, Medicare hospital expenditures grew by 270 percent. Between 1975 and 1983, they grew by 250 percent (U.S. Department of Health and Human Services, 1984).

The experience with hospital reimbursement during this initial era of Medicare's history offers several important lessons. When the method of reimbursement creates undesirable forms of behavior, it will be difficult to design a regulatory system that does more than partially suppress them. Consequently, to effectively deal with rising costs Congress needed to revise its reimbursement practices. This would take Medicare outside the mainstream of American medical care, as private insurers continued to pay providers on the basis of cost (or, even more generously, on the basis of charges).

Incentives and Performance in the 1980s

By the early 1980s, the continued growth of hospital expenditures and the antiregulatory political mood in Washington, D.C. made it clear that changes were needed in the way Medicare paid hospitals. A series of amendments were enacted, culminating in Medicare's current Prospective Payment System (PPS).

Hospital reimbursement provisions were initially altered by the Omnibus Budget Reconciliation Act of 1981 (OBRA) and the Tax Equity and Fiscal Responsibility Act (TEFRA) of 1982. OBRA limited reimbursements for a variety of inpatient and outpatient services and TEFRA established a flat price per patient based on the historic average costs of care in the hospital. In combination, the 1981 and 1982 programs imposed the equivalent of hospital budget caps for Medicare patients (provided there was no expansion in either bed capacity or percentage of Medicare patients treated at the hospital).

These reforms were seen as threatening by the hospital industry because they paid for care almost entirely based on average cost with few adjustments for legitimate variations in hospital expenses due to severity of patients' illness. Partly as a result of efforts led by the hospital industry, these hospital-payment provisions were short lived, overridden by Title VI of the Social Security amendments of 1983 that created Medicare's PPS.

The prospective payment system pays hospitals on the basis of a predetermined price per admission. The goal of the program is to establish a uniform national set of prices for 468 different *categories of diagnoses*. Hospitals are paid for each patient based on the Diagnosis-Related Group (DRG) into which he or she is categorized. These payments are adjusted for the average wage rate in the hospital's community, its rural or urban location and whether it is a teaching hospital. Extremely long stays are designated as outliers and are reimbursed on the basis of costs.[2]

This approach was preferred to TEFRA by the hospital industry because it reflected at least to some extent differences in case mix among hospitals. Because historically there have been large regional differences in hospital expenses, though, there was concern that national prices would lead to disruptively large transfers of Medicare dollars from high- to low-cost regions (Vladeck, 1985). Consequently, national rates were to be phased in over a four-year period to allow hospitals time to adjust. In the interim, DRG payments were based in part on national average cost for each DRG, in part on regional average costs and in part on the hospital's historic costs.

Incentives Created Under DRGs

Prospective payment using DRGs creates very different incentives than does cost-based reimbursement, and it represents a significant shift along the efficiency-access trade-off. Instead of promoting utilization, at the cost of waste and inefficiency, PPS encourages efficiency at the risk of inadequate provision of services. Because DRGs set a price in advance for each admission, hospitals have an incentive to conserve the services and personnel used to treat patients and to reduce length of stay (Kuntz, 1984; Richards, 1984; U.S. Congress, Office of Technology Assessment, 1985), even though they may in the process provide too few services or discharge patients who are too sick to be adequately cared for in nonhospital settings (Newcomer et al., 1985).

The prospective payment system may not in practice create as much efficiency as initially hoped. Paying a hospital per admission encourages hospitals to increase the number of patients they treat. Hospitals can profit by repeatedly discharging and admitting the same patients to maximize revenues. The average hospitalized elder has six pathological conditions (Rowe, 1985). Instead of treating these simultaneously, the hospital may choose to treat them sequentially.

DRGs will almost certainly reduce access to hospital services. The current prospective payment system creates incentives for hospitals to discourage admission of patients who are relatively expensive to treat within each DRG (Berenson and Pawlson, 1984). Under PPS hospitals also have an incentive to specialize. As Richard S. Schweiker, then secretary of the Department of Health and Human Services (DHHS), predicted when he introduced PPS legislation to Congress, "Hospitals may tend to expand in areas [types of services] in which they can provide care more efficiently than other hospitals and to contract in those areas where they are relatively less efficient. . . . No longer will most hospitals be able to supply all forms of specialized care" (1982, pp. 102–3).[3] Medicare beneficiaries with specialized needs may thus no longer be able to obtain care at the hospital nearest their home. Because distance to a hospital is an important determinant of access for elders with limited mobility, this may make it more difficult for them to obtain needed services (Inguanzo and Harju, 1985).

As a check on the incentives for multiple admissions and premature discharges, a new federal utilization review system was put in place. Peer Review Organizations (PROs) were created to replace PSROs and charged with reviewing the medical necessity, appropriateness, quality and cost-effectiveness of care received by Medicare beneficiaries. In their initial contracts, PROs were directed to focus on readmissions, "largely for cost-containment purposes" (U.S. Congress, Office of Technology Assessment, 1985, p. 83).

Access, Costs and Quality Under PPS

It is difficult at this time to provide more than a sketchy assessment of the effects of Medicare's shift to PPS. The DRGs are still being phased in, so that the full incentives have yet to be felt by providers (Guterman and Dobson, 1986). Because hospitals will require time to adjust to these incentives, changes in behavior are not likely to be fully evident for several years (U.S. Congress, Office of Technology Assessment, 1985). A number of facilities, including psychiatric hospitals, children's hospitals and sole community hospitals are fully or partially exempted from the system. Enough evidence has accumulated, however, to conclude that the PPS is producing some of the expected effects but not others.

Increases in Medicare's spending on hospital care have dramatically slowed, apparently at least in part owing to incentives produced by DRGs. In 1984, the real costs of hospital care for Medicare enrollees grew at half the rate it had in 1983 and a third of the rate at which costs had increased between 1975 and 1982 (Guterman and Dobson, 1986). Much of this slowing was produced by a large drop in elders' average length of stay, which fell twice as fast as it had in recent years (Guterman and Dobson, 1986).[4] Surprisingly, some of the cost savings came from a reduction in hospital admissions, though it had been predicted that DRGs would stimulate more admissions. This unexpected decline has been attributed to the shock factor of confronting doctors and hospitals with a radically different payment system (Davis et al., 1985).

It is too early to definitively assess the impact of PPS on quality, but preliminary evidence suggests that the same incentives that have increased efficiency are leading to less-adequate treatment. Surveys indicate that about half of all hospital administrators and two thirds of physicians feel that PPS has compromised care within the facility (Glenn and Brazda, 1985a, 1985c).[5]

Premature discharge of medicare patients is seen as a particularly pressing problem. The inspector general of DHHS documented 3,700 cases considered to be prematurely discharged or inappropriately transferred among facilities between mid-1984 and mid-1985. Half of the respondents on a survey of internal medicine specialists during the same period reported that they had been pressured to discharge patients early; 40 percent of these thought that this adversely affected beneficiaries' health (Glenn and Brazda, 1985c). Surveys conducted in 1986 by the American Medical Association found that 48 percent of American physicians reported that they felt "unduly pressured" to discharge Medicare patients early from the hospital (Harvey, 1986).

There is even less evidence about the effects of PPS on access to hospital care. Although health professionals had expected that "patients may find it more difficult to get the full range of services and conveniences that many have come to expect" (Arthur Anderson and Co., 1984, p. 18), there is little empirical evidence supporting this prediction. A staff report by the Senate Committee on Aging, released in September 1985, did find some cases in which elders with multiple medical problems were denied admission to a hospital. About 10 percent of complaints lodged with the office of the Massachusetts state ombudsman involved alleged denial of admission (Barnes, 1986).

Somewhat unexpectedly, the most adverse effects of DRGs on access to medical services seem to come for patients *after* they leave the hospital. Because prospective payment encourages quicker discharge of patients from the hospital, they tend to be sicker and more difficult for nursing homes and home health care agencies to treat. Some agencies lack the capacity to adapt to these sicker patients. Others lack the financial resources. Because Medicare reimburses based on historic costs, which were generated by treating a healthier set of elders, reimbursement to nursing homes and home health agencies may be inadequate to cover the costs of the sickest elders. In a survey conducted by the General Accounting Office in 1986, 79% of responding hospital discharge planners reported that Medicare's prospective payment system had made it more difficult to place patients in post-hospital settings in 1985, compared to 1982 (U.S. General Accounting Office, 1987).

Because almost all these assessments of quality and access are based on respondents' perceptions rather than objective clinical measures, it is difficult to determine their reliability and even harder to assess the extent to which problems are due to the incentives produced by PPS as opposed to other ongoing changes in the health care system. Nonetheless, it seems likely that Medicare's DRG system creates, as would any form of prospective payment, incentives that both encourage efficiency and that lead to financial pressures to limit treatment and discourage access to care.

Options for dealing with these undesirable consequences will be discussed later in the chapter.

To assess the long-term effects of DRGs it is useful to consider the experience of New Jersey, which has used DRGs to set hospital payments since the late 1970s. The evidence from preliminary studies suggests that employing a DRG-based payment system does not ensure effective cost containment. Findings indicated that costs were reduced to only a limited extent (Health Research and Educational Trust of New Jersey, 1984) in part because length of stay in hospitals did not decline significantly (May and Wasserman, 1984). Later research established that DRGs produced some cost savings per admission but that these were partially offset by increased admissions (Hsiao et al., 1986; Rosko and Broyles, 1986).

New Jersey's system, however, differs from Medicare's in several important ways. In New Jersey, hospitals received increased allowances for such items as depreciation, bad debts and working capital. Furthermore, the New Jersey payment system provided generous exceptions for high-cost patients and paid hospitals only in part based on patient DRGs; reimbursement was determined in part by the hospitals' historic costs. As a result, the basis for payment was, in actuality, mostly the hospital's own costs, not a normative standard cost.

The New Jersey experience did identify two practical problems with the DRG approach. First, important factors such as patients' health status and severity of illness were not adequately taken into account by DRGs. Second, using DRGs as a measure of hospital case mix creates incentives as well as opportunities for hospitals to game the system by strategically labeling patients with particular diagnoses in order to maximize hospital reimbursement. These shortcomings are examples of a more general issue, or trade-off, that exists under any prospective payment system. Prospective payment rates must strike a balance between low rates (which would be appropriate for healthier patients, but too low for the more severely ill) and high rates (which would be appropriate for the sickest patients, but overpay providers for all others). As a result, providers are overpaid for treating relatively healthy patients, but underpaid for treating the most severely ill Medicare beneficiaries.

An Emerging Trade-off: Equity Versus Administrability

Any prospective payment system must deal with a trade-off between administrability and equitable treatment of patients and providers. If the reimbursement system is to treat individual patients and hospitals fairly, its prices must be set in a way that recognizes legitimate differences in costs of treatment (Ellis, 1986). Grouping patients by diagnosis was intended to accomplish this. "These DRGs are used to classify patients into groups that are clinically coherent and homogeneous with respect to resource use. Such a classification scheme allows for equitable payment across hospitals in that comparable services can be comparably remunerated" (Guterman and Dobson, 1986, pp. 97).

Certainly DRGs do this more effectively than did the reimbursement system proposed in TEFRA. Nonetheless, costs of treating patients are affected by a variety of characteristics of the patient, the hospital and the community in which they are located. Hospital payments under PPS reflect only some of these factors. Introducing more factors into the reimbursement formula would avoid underpaying some cases while overpaying others. It would also, however, add to the complexity of the program.

For example, grouping patients into over 400 DRG categories accounts for only some of the differences in complexity of illness. DRGs explain at most only a third of the difference between high- and low-cost surgical cases and considerably less for medical diagnoses (Taube et al., 1984). No one envisions that the remaining differences in costs among patients are due entirely to differences in efficiency; at least half seem to be associated with differences in severity of illness that are not measured by DRGs (Horn et al., 1984).

Similarly, there are significant differences in characteristics of hospitals that are not reflected by DRGs. PPS does include special adjustments for facilities located in areas that are urban or that have a high cost of living. An additional adjustment is made for hospitals with teaching affiliations. In spite of these refinements, PPS is predicted to produce a major redistribution of resources among hospitals (Vaida, 1984; U.S. Congress, Office of Technology Assessment, 1985) that is only partially related to differences in operating efficiency (American Hospital Association, 1984).

These examples illustrate a fundamental design issue in any prospective payment system: To treat patients and providers more equitably the system must inevitably become more complex. The more complex the system, the more difficult it is to administer.

The current PPS was designed to balance the goals of equity and administrability. As with all compromises, it is fully satisfying to no one. On the one hand, it seems too complicated. By establishing a large number of payment categories, the system creates a number of perverse incentives. For example, providers have an incentive to reclassify patients into DRGs that are most profitable (Jencks et al., 1984). There is great latitude for this DRG creep in the elderly because so many enter a hospital with multiple pathologies. Studies suggest that there have, in fact, been reclassification of patients toward more-complex (and more highly reimbursable) diagnoses (Guterman and Dobson, 1986).

On the other hand, the system appears to some to be too simplistic. By setting a single national rate for each DRG, it will encourage massive redistributions of resources from the West and upper Midwest to the South and Southeast (Vaida, 1984; Vladeck, 1985). The simple distinctions between urban and rural hospitals inadequately reflect the variations in costs faced by facilities located in large metropolitan areas (Porter, 1984).

These problems are not unique to Medicare's current PPS. Any prospective payment system must strike a balance between the goals of equity and administrability. In doing so, every system will in turn be criticized as being too complex, too simplistic or both. It is too soon to determine whether or not PPS has struck the "right" balance, but a number of reforms have been proposed to move the system in either one direction or the other.

Options for Medicare Hospital Reimbursement Reform

Proposed changes in the way that Medicare pays for hospital care fall into two broad categories: those that supplement or modify the existing DRG system and those that replace DRGs with some other system for setting prices.

Modifications to DRGs address a number of the problems discussed earlier.

Proposals include additional adjustments to reflect specific characteristics of patients and providers, administrative innovations to preserve quality and accessibility of care and the linking of Medicare's payment rates to those of other payers to encourage greater efficiency and equity.

Alternatives to DRGs strike a different balance among the goals of efficiency, access, equity and administrability. Some approaches, for example, calculate reimbursement as a mix, or blend, of prospective and cost-based rates. This reduces incentives for efficiency, but it more completely reflects legitimate differences in costs among hospitals. Other proposals would have Medicare set budgets or budget targets for hospitals instead of setting prices. This provides more complete control of cost, but it may also create greater pressures to limit access to care if the hospital spends more than its budget in a given year.[6]

Modifications in the DRG System

Fine-Tuning DRGs

As noted, the current DRG system does not measure the resource needs for treating different patients. As a result, a number of modifications to DRGs have been proposed, some based on characteristics of patients, others on characteristics of hospitals.

It is generally accepted that DRGs do not adequately account for differences in severity of illness among patients. As a result, DRG payments are too low to pay for the care of the sickest patients, thus creating a financial incentive for hospitals to avoid admitting or to prematurely discharge these beneficiaries (Gertman and Lowenstein, 1984). A number of approaches incorporate more accurate measures of patients' health into the DRG system. These include measures of "disease staging" (e.g., how advanced the illness is when first treated), "patient management" (e.g., how complex the treatment process is) and "severity of illness" (e.g,, how medically complicated the illness is) (Jencks et al., 1984).

Any of these measures incorporated into DRGs provides additional information about the patient and therefore better predicts needed treatment costs than do DRGs alone. Adding to the complexity of patient classification under PPS, however, also has some serious drawbacks.

First, more categories add considerably to the complexity of the system. This imposes costs on both the Medicare program and hospitals. The more categories there are, the more difficult it is for federal administrators to determine how new technologies or techniques alter the categories into which patients should be placed. The New Jersey experience suggests that this can be done far more expeditiously with fewer categories; some reviews of New Jersey's DRG system suggested that "the number of DRGS should be reduced in order to make the method easier to administer" (Grimaldi, 1981).

Hospitals have put considerable resources into adapting to DRG-based reimbursement. Many believe that this has improved their managerial capabilities, though this remains a topic of debate (Packer, 1985; Hsiao et al., 1986). Adding yet more categories, however, would add to the costs of understanding and responding to reimbursement incentives. It might also make it difficult for hospital administrators to use the reimbursement classifications as information for management purposes because they would have too few patients admitted within each category to determine if their hospitals' performance matched national standards (Jencks et al., 1984).

Second, the more complex the classification scheme, the more complicated and in some cases inappropriate, will be the incentives it creates. Introducing additional categories may make it more difficult to determine if hospital administrators are reclassifying patients into more remunerative payment groups (Grimaldi, 1981). Reimbursing for severity of illness may actually lead to incentives for providers to delay treatment of an illness to increase reimbursement (Gertman and Lowenstein, 1984).

Finally, because there are many plausible schemes for fine-tuning DRGs, political pressures may increasingly complicate and fragment Medicare's PPS.[7] No single system is likely to prove preferable on technical grounds or for all beneficiaries. Some approaches will prove more lucrative for certain types of hospitals, others more profitable for different hospitals. Under these circumstances, each set of hospitals will lobby for a different severity-of-illness measure. As a result, hospital reimbursement for different diagnoses, different parts of the country or different medical specialities might be fine-tuned in different ways, making PPS more complex, confusing and difficult to monitor.

A second approach to adjusting DRGs incorporates additional characteristics of the hospital. For example, during the past several years, there has been a debate raging in Washington over whether Medicare should more generously reimburse so-called disproportionate-share hospitals—those that treat a large share of low-income patients. Congress has authorized special compensation several times, yet DHHS has balked at this change.

There is no disagreement that caring for Medicare patients in these hospitals has historically been more costly than in the average hospital (American Hospital Association, 1984). The question is whether these costs reflect legitimate differences in health care needs or inefficiency in the facility. The American Hospital Association (AHA) takes the first position. In contrast, in a recently formulated report, "HHS concludes that disproportionate share hospitals do have higher than average costs, but finds the reasons for this to be unclear. HHS tentatively attributes the cost differences to inefficient management, higher overhead and labor expenses, and more severely ill patients" (Glenn and Brazda, 1985b).

Whatever the merits of the two sides in this particular debate, it illustrates a more general issue that will continue to arise under prospective payment: Which cost differences among facilities are legitimate and, therefore, should be covered in payment rates? Which should be eliminated? Costs in hospitals are affected to some extent by their perceived mission, that is, by their institutional goals. By incorporating some types of cost differences but not others, a prospective payment system legitimizes certain types of hospital policies but makes others financially infeasible.

For example, not all hospitals have the same opportunities to reduce cost through specialization; some have missions that require them to admit a full spectrum of patients. Teaching hospitals must treat patients with a variety of conditions to educate their students effectively. Public hospitals are charged with the responsibility of caring for all patients who present themselves for treatment (Brown, 1983).[8] As a result, neither type of facility can fully pursue opportunities for specialization, and their costs will consequently be higher than those of other hospitals (Marmor et al., 1986).[9] The public good might not be served, however, by forcing them to eliminate these higher costs through specialization.

More generally, hospitals serve a variety of functions in the community that may increase their costs, such as providing needed, but uninsured, services or offering very-high-quality treatment. In an increasingly competitive environment, it will become more difficult for hospitals to play this role unless adequately reimbursed (Sigmond, 1985). If a prospective payment system does not incorporate a mechanism for identifying and paying for costs incurred in these broader social roles, hospitals' orientation to the special needs of their community may well disappear as a result of homogenizing payment arrangements. How these legitimate functions are best identified is unclear, but it is not a determination that can be based on purely technical considerations, nor should it be made without appropriate public input.

Administrative and Regulatory Reforms

When Medicare's cost-based reimbursement encouraged overutilization and inefficiency, attempts were made, with moderate success, to address these issues through administrative mechanisms like PSROs and CON. Now that PPS creates incentives for undertreatment and for discouraging access, proposals have been made for new regulatory approaches to control these problems.

To address concerns about inadequate treatment and premature discharge Congress has charged PROs with increased responsibility for ensuring that beneficiaries receive adequate care. Although the principle goal for PROs when first established in 1984 was reducing Medicare admissions, by the summer of 1985, the Health Care Financing Administration (HCFA) announced that it would include more quality-of-care criteria in awarding PRO contracts and was experimenting with concurrent review of hospital transfers (Glenn and Brazda, 1985a & c). Some in Congress have called for an even more pronounced shift in goals. Representative Edward R. Roybal, chairman of the House Select Committee on Aging, has proposed requiring that PROs devote 50 percent of their resources to quality assurance.

It is unclear how effective this approach will be. For many cases, there simply are not clear professional standards for hospitalization or treatment (Gertman and Lowenstein, 1985). As a result, it may prove quite difficult to identify inappropriate or inadequate treatment. This is particularly true for chronic illness, which is very common among the elderly. For a chronically impaired beneficiary, the most important determinants of appropriate treatment may be social or economic rather than medical (Rowe, 1985). A review board composed of physicians and using medical criteria may thus not provide a very effective review of quality of care.

PROs may also not have sufficiently broad oversight to truly ensure adequate quality of care for beneficiaries. DRGs have encouraged hospitals to shift to outpatient settings a number of procedures that previously had been performed in the hospital (U.S. Congress, Office of Technology Assessment, 1985). In addition, as discussed earlier, some of the most important adverse effects of DRGs may befall elders who are denied admission to the hospital or who have difficulty obtaining care once they are discharged from the hospital. But PROs remain focused on hospitals. As a result of this narrow purview, the adequacy of much of the care received by elders goes unmonitored by PROs.

An alternative approach, complementary to review by PROs, would identify the problems of quality and accessibility of services as perceived by beneficiaries. Currently, complaints about refusals of admission are being handled by a national hot line set up by DHHS and, in some states, by a designated health ombudsmen. If current problems grow, however, it may prove necessary to decentralize this process and establish local or regional offices for handling beneficiaries' concerns.

Barriers to access are not created solely by restrictions established by providers. If beneficiaries do not fully understand their Medicare coverage or their options for treatment, they may fail to seek the most appropriate care. As discussed in Chapter 4, beneficiaries have traditionally relied on providers, particularly hospital discharge planners, to provide them with the necessary information. The incentives embodied in PPS, however, may create situations in which the interests of the hospital and the beneficiary are not identical. Under these circumstances, the hospital can no longer be viewed as a reliable source of information. A recent report by the Senate Aging Committee documented a number of cases in which elders were misinformed by hospitals about their coverage. Other reports have found similar problems:

> Many elders express concern as to whether their physician will present a good case for their hospitalization. . . . In addition to a high level of ignorance as to the admission and treatment process under DRGs, a similar lack of knowledge exists concerning the appeals process, primarily because there is little attempt made by hospital admitting personnel and discharge planners to explain to the patient his or her rights under the appeals process (Kerschner, 1986, p. 31).

In the last year, hospitals have been required to read Medicare patients a bill of rights when admitted. This offers only limited information and may not provide the information elders require at the time decisions about treatment are being made. It may, therefore, be necessary to establish an office that assumes a more active role in providing elders with information and in following up on their complaints. Such an ombudsman office could be based in local Social Security or Administration on Aging offices. It could serve a primary function of providing beneficiaries with information and a secondary function of collecting evidence on problems of access emerging in the PPS.

Such a proposal, however, might encounter some resistance. It creates a new public agency at a time when there are political pressures to cut bureaucracy, and adds to the costs of the Medicare program. These costs would not be particularly large—based on the record of similar efforts at the state level, a minimal program might require $15 million to $20 million annually. These would be costs, though, that do not yield any direct benefit in terms of health care services. Programs with only indirect benefits are traditionally difficult to fund in an era of constrained federal budgets.

Establishing All-Payers Reimbursement Systems

Medicare was the first major insurance program to adopt prospective payment using DRGs. Being first has certain disadvantages. Hospitals that treat only a small number of Medicare patients may not be adequately motivated to respond to the incentives created by DRGs. If the federal govenment continues to restrict the annual increase in reimbursement rates, Medicare beneficiaries will become progressively less profitable to treat than are other patients and hospitals may be tempted to discourage the admission of elders in favor of more profitable, privately insured patients.

To meet these concerns it has been proposed (by Senator Edward M. Kennedy and Representative Richard A. Gephardt) that Medicare and other payers use a single unified payment system. Several states (Maine, Maryland, Massachusetts, New Jersey, and New York) have adopted such all-payers systems. Under these arrangements, rates among payers are either equalized or any differences are based on differences in the costs of treating patients or processing claims for the various payors (Meyer, 1986).

This unified approach has several advantages over the disparate payment arrangements that now prevail throughout most of the country. First, it creates consistent incentives to which hospitals can respond—institutions are no longer faced by a plethora of payment schemes with a host of conflicting incentives (Hsiao et al., 1986). Second, it ensures that reimbursement rates across payers stay in line with one another. This reduces the propensity to discriminate against patients according to their source of payment.[10] Finally, an all-payers system provides an institutional mechanism through which private and public insurers can agree to pay a "fair share" of the cost of treating the uninsured (Wilensky, 1986).

Although such a system would be complicated to establish, the experience of the states that have adopted an all-payers approach proves it is feasible. An all-payers system need not be limited to DRG-based reimbursement; it could be adapted to any system of prospective payment.[11] Most proponents agree that such systems should be implemented on the state level; past state-level experience can serve as a guide (much as the New Jersey experience provided a guide for Medicare DRGs).

There are, however, a number of obstacles to developing an all-payers system. It requires a more extensive system of rate regulation than now exists. Regulatory approaches are not in political favor and all-payers systems have been attacked by using the same arguments traditionally made against regulation generally:

> Even if one favors the programmatic concepts adopted by all-payers systems, however, one could oppose the hospital rate-setting apparatus that has been inextricably bound up with these provisions . . . a regulatory device is not likely to provide a mechanism for separating waste from need. . . . Ironically, most of these regulatory measures are actually roadblocks to long-term cost relief, as they stifle potential cost-saving innovations and protect inefficiency" (Meyer, 1986, 178–79).

Though it covers more parties, it is unclear that an all-payers system is any more regulatory than are DRGs alone; the latter system is itself a form of detailed rate setting. The DRGs were sold politically, however, as a procompetitive measure, encouraging hospitals to compete to get patients at a preestablished price (Schweiker, 1982). Certainly if DRGs foster competition, an all-payers system would do so to an even greater degree by creating a level playing field on which hospitals could compete for public and private patients.

The second barrier to establishing an all-payers system stems from the fact that it requires cooperation from Medicare, Medicaid, Blue Cross and commercial insurers. The prevailing trends in health insurance favor competition rather than cooperation. Both Medicaid and private insurers are increasingly turning to preferred provider arrangements in which they contract with selected hospitals and physician groups (Rice et al., 1985). The competitive dynamic involves each payer seeking the best deal available, and this goal may conflict with efforts to strike fair deals for all payers.

The obstacles to creating a unified system, though, become smaller if most or all payers are already using a similar method of paying hospitals. It seems likely that DRGs will provide this common ground. Already several states have adopted DRGs for their Medicaid programs. It is the opinion of many health professionals that DRGs will be the system of choice for both public and private insurers in the 1990s (Arthur Andersen and Co., 1984). If this occurs, it would facilitate the creation of DRG-based all-payers systems in the future.

Finally, although under some circumstances the creation of uniform incentives for hospitals is an advantage of all-payers systems, this may not always be true. As we have discussed, DRGs create incentives for behavior that are both socially desirable (increased efficiency) and socially undesirable (restrictions on access and reductions in quality). When only Medicare uses DRGs, hospitals may be less likely to go through the administrative effort to reduce waste, but they will also be less likely to identify and adopt admissions criteria that screen out the unprofitable patients in each DRG. With an all-payers system, however, the incentives currently created by Medicare's DRGs will be felt more strongly by hospitals. If it proves difficult to adopt administrative or other reforms to limit these undesirable side effects, it may not be advantageous to reinforce DRG-based incentives. Because any method of prospective payment will lead to some problematic outcomes, this concern applies to any type of all-payers system.

Alternatives to DRG-Based Reimbursement

Mixed Reimbursement Systems

As we have seen, DRGs may create some undesirable incentives. But these shortcomings are by no means limited to DRG-based reimbursement. Any prospective payment system, by pressuring the hospital to cut costs, may lead to reductions in quality as well as waste, to cutting muscle as well as fat. Because of these limitations, some observers have advocated that Medicare's reimbursement should be based only partly on prospective rates and partly based on hospitals' historic costs. These mixed systems are designed to moderate the constraints on quality and access produced by pure prospective payment.

Mixed systems can combine prospective and retrospective payment in two different ways. The first combines the two when calculating the rates at which hospitals are paid. Under these arrangements, payment for a given patient in a hospital might be based partially on national rates for that patient's DRG and partially on the hospital's historic costs (Ellis and McGuire, 1986). Adopting the term used by the AHA, we will refer to this approach as a *blended reimbursement system.*[12] The second mixed system pays some hospitals or pays for some types of patients by using prospective payment and pays others by using cost-based reimbursement. We will refer to this as a *side-by-side reimbursement system.*

Each of these mixed approaches is already a part of Medicare's PPS. Sole community hospitals are paid using rates based one-quarter on the regional DRG rate and three-quarters on historic costs. Psychiatric hospitals (and designated psychiatric units in general hospitals), children's hospitals and chronic-care hospitals are all still paid on the basis of costs rather than DRGs. The intent of Congress, as expressed in the legislation first authorizing DRGs, was that eventually prospective payment would become the sole standard of reimbursement. Thus the question is whether this sort of standardization makes sense or whether mixed reimbursement should be preserved or even expanded.

One of the principal proponents of blended reimbursement has been the AHA. In their proposed system, the extent to which each DRG is set prospectively rather than cost-based would depend on the size of the variance in costs among hospitals for that DRG. When the distribution of costs is narrow, rates would be set almost entirely prospectively; when the variance is large, payment would be based mainly on the hospital's historic costs (American Hospital Association, 1984). This blending is similar to the method by which New Jersey has calculated its DRG reimbursement rates.

Blending in this way is claimed to have a number of advantages. It is argued to be more equitable to hospitals. Blending, the AHA suggests, could do away with the need for urban/rural and disporportionate-share adjustments and simplify what is viewed as a patchwork system. At the same time, blending is thought to preserve the incentives for efficiency produced by prospective payment because all DRGs would be at least in part prospectively determined:

> DRG-specific price blending is just a more equitable and realistic way of moving to national rates. For those DRGs whose cost distributions are wide, the move will be more evolutionary, reflecting clinical realities. . . . DRG-specific price blending also preserves the incentives built into the current PPS . . . all hospitals will have the incentive to keep their costs per case below the blended national average/institution-specific rates as well as keep the annual rate of increase in their costs per case below the national rate of increase in prices" (American Hospital Association, 1984, pp. 4–5).

Some early research, based on computer simulation models, indicates that a mixed system of this type would in fact be more equitable for providers and possibly for patients (Ellis, 1986; Siegel et al., 1986). These are important benefits and are likely to produce indirect benefits of greater access and quality of care. There are likely to be, however, some disadvantages as well.

First, blending will reduce the incentives for greater efficiency (Hsiao et al., 1986). Hospitals paid under blended DRGs in New Jersey reduced both costs and length of stay less than did hospitals paid with Medicare DRGs (May and Wasserman, 1984; Guterman and Dobson, 1986). Second, blending will almost certainly add to the administrative burden on the system. Even if urban/rural distinctions and the like were eliminated, blending replaces a system using adjustments for a small number of classes of hospitals with one in which HCFA must calculate a separate set of rates for every individual facility. This would force HCFA to maintain its traditional bureaucracy to determine what constitutes legitimate costs for cost-based reimbursement in addition to the bureaucracy necessary to administer prospective payments.

Finally, it is unclear that the proportion of prospective and cost-based rates should be based on the observed interhospital variation in costs. Although this variance very likely reflects a lack of clinical consensus on the treatment of illness, it is probably the case that those illnesses with less clearly defined treatment protocols are those for which there is the greatest unnecessary utilization (Wennberg et al., 1984). By disproportionately reducing the cost-saving incentives for these DRGs, one may well eliminate much of the potential for cutting waste from the hospital system.

Side-by-side reimbursement systems address the inadequacies of DRGs by simply exempting certain diagnoses or facilities from the PPS. This has the advantage of administrative simplicity, but it removes entirely any incentives for greater efficiency for those diagnoses that remain reimbursed on the basis of costs.

Moreover, by paying some facilities on the basis of costs, the system encourages providers to shift resources to those facilities because they can avoid dealing with the financial pressures and administrative burdens of prospective payment. Over the past several years, for example, many hospital corporations have moved their investments from short-term general hospitals to psychiatric institutions (Levenson, 1985; Schlesinger, 1985). Because the diagnoses that are likely to be exempted from prospective payment are those for which there is the least clinical consensus on treatment, there is considerable potential for providers to induce demand, thus adding to their revenues and increasing Medicare expenditures (Wennberg et al., 1984).

Prospective Budgets and Budget Targets

Medicare's PPS represents an attempt to control costs by controlling prices. This will be effective only if providers have little discretion over the volume of services or if their behavior can be effectively monitored and controlled through some form of utilization review. Evidence accumulated over the past several decades, though, suggests that most clinical decision making is highly discretionary (Wennberg, 1983). Lack of consensus leads to geographic variation in per capita admission rates, in procedures performed per admission, and in decisions about whether and where to perform outpatient surgery. Under these circumstances, there is considerable leeway for hospitals to encourage additional admissions to make up for revenue lost if prices are controlled (Wennberg et al., 1984). It is difficult to limit these responses through utilization review (Dans et al., 1985).

The past performance of hospital rate-regulation systems documents this problem (Sloan, 1983; Eby and Cohodes, 1985). Medicare's 1972 cap on so-called routine costs of hospital services under Section 223 led to a proliferation of laboratory and other ancillary services in the subsequent years. Attempts by states to limit hospital per diem rates have led to increases in lengths of stay and admissions (Worthington and Piro, 1982). Evidence from New Jersey—where DRGs apply to all payers and have been in place long enough to affect physician practice patterns—indicates that the per capita admission rates have risen there as well (Hsiao et al., 1986; Rosko and Broyles, 1986).

Medicare's hospital expenditures can be effectively limited only if price *and volume* are constrained. One way to do this is to set a budget or budget target for each hospital's spending on Medicare beneficiaries. Budget targets involve establishing a prespecified level of expenditure either on a hospital-by-hospital or regional basis. Facilities (or regions) that kept annual costs below their target would receive some incentive payment (i.e., a portion of the savings). Hospitals exceeding their target would face a financial penalty. Massachusetts, operating under a law called Chapter 372, has shown that such a system of budget-based incentives is administratively feasible.[13]

Budget allocations provide each hospital with a predetermined amount of money to use in treating patients. In its simplest form, this approach imposes an absolute budget cap on the facility (though if year-end adjustments are permitted, the incentives may be very similar to those of a system based on target budgets). Budget allocations have been a part of the Canadian national health insurance system since the late 1960s.

There is little doubt that budgetary constraints can control costs. Chapter 372 significantly decreased the growth of hospital costs in Massachusetts; the lower rate of increase in hospital expenditures has remained stable since the law was enacted in 1982 at a level comparable to the nationwide experience with DRGs (Carter, 1986).[14] Budgetary allocations contained costs in Canada, even in a system with little patient copayment. Hospital expenditures throughout the 1970s and 1980s grew more slowly in that country than in the United States (Evans, 1985). A study of the province of Ontario concluded, for example, that "it appears that global budgeting may have been moderately successful in controlling hospital cost inflation in Ontario. . . . From 1972 to 1980–81, total expenditures in all Ontario hospitals grew by 29 percent over and above general inflation, compared to 54 percent in the United States" (Detsky et al., 1983, p. 156). Because cost per admission rose at roughly the same rate in both countries, most of the savings came from reduced utilization.

At the same time, compared to DRGs, budget constraints are relatively nonintrusive from both clinical and administrative points of view. Physicians and hospital administrators would have great latitude in making clinical and administrative decisions within the budget, perhaps enhancing quality.

By creating more comprehensive controls on hospital costs, however, budget-based reimbursement may also have some undesirable side effects. By limiting total expenditures, it forces providers to choose, to some extent, between admitting additional Medicare patients and providing more treatment for those admitted. Because undertreatment of patients already in the hospital is more visible and more readily regulated than is a policy to discourage admissions, budget targets may lead to inappropriately restricted access.

Prospective budgeting would also encourage the shift of services to outpatient settings. Although past studies have shown that outpatients care is, case by case, less expensive than comparable inpatient care, this shift may also lead to increases in utilization of outpatient services that are sufficient to increase overall costs.

Although conceptually simple, the ease and cost of administration of budget caps depend largely on the manner in which they are implemented. A cap at a regional level would be more easily administered by the federal government, perhaps through HCFA's existing regional offices.

A state-by-state cap, however, could take advantage of existing state experience with hospital rate regulation. States would also be in the best position to establish all-payers arrangements using budgets. States have legal responsibility for regulating the health insurance industry and have experience in doing so. States have the authority to establish Medicaid payment rates; they would, therefore, have to participate in any all-payers budgeting system in any case. Allowing states discretion in adopting all-payers systems permits design of systems that are more responsive to local needs and conditions than a nationally uniform system like the current Medicare PPS. It would, though, lead to greater state rather than federal influence on resource-allocation decisions. The checkered history of the Medicaid program suggests caution in introducing states as partners in a federal program such as Medicare (Davidson et al., 1986).

Finally, any budget-based system creates an important, though subtle, change in the orientation of the Medicare program. If hospital budgets are truly fixed, the program no longer offers true "entitlement" to treatment; it becomes a quasi entitlement like that in the Veterans Administration health care system (Schlesinger et al., 1984). This could have important political ramifications for the program, because beneficiaries are being asked to pay a lifetime of payroll taxes for uncertain future benefits. These problems could be lessened, to some extent, by using budget targets (which rely on budget-based incentives) rather than budget caps (which fix the total pool of resources).

Political Feasibility for PPS Reform

The challenge that the Medicare program will face in the next decade is to establish a hospital reimbursement policy that appropriately balances conflicting goals. Partially as a response to the excesses of the past, much of today's debate over the Medicare program focuses on cost containment and the elimination of unnecessary utilization. These are important policy objectives, but so is the provision of acceptable, equitable health care services to Medicare's beneficiaries. In the future refinement of prospective hospital reimbursement, the program must also balance program simplicity and administrative ease against equitable treatment of patients and providers.

This balancing act effort will probably be undertaken using a DRG-based reimbursement system. For several reasons, we expect that DRGs will remain Medicare's method of paying hospitals, at least in the near future. The DRGs are given much of the credit in Washington for recent reductions in the growth of hospital expenses for the elderly (Sullivan, 1985). Although popular perceptions probably overstate their role—a number of other ongoing trends, including the growth of HMOs and expansion of outpatient surgery facilities, also have contributed to lower rates of hospitalization (Davis et al., 1985)—it seems very likely that DRGs, like earlier state-based prospective payment systems, will cut the annual inflation of hospital costs by a few percentage points. Understandably, Congress will be slow to abandon a system that seems to be working.

In addition, there are important advantages to maintaining a stable payment system. Hospitals have spent considerable resources identifying and adapting to the incentives created by DRGs. Only now, four years after the program was enacted, are we gaining some sense of the consequences of DRGs for access and quality of care. To shift in the near future to an entirely new method of payment would force everyone to take up the learning process from the start. If the basis of Medicare's reimbursement system is continually changing, it will be difficult for providers to develop any reliable long-term strategies, thus hindering their ability to innovate administratively or to develop new services.

Consequently, in the short term it is probably most reasonable to think in terms of fine-tuning DRGs to provide for greater equity or better protections for access and quality of care. A number of alternatives for doing this were described earlier. In addition, the basic DRG system might be modified to become an all-payers DRG system or one that uses blended pricing based in part on DRGs.

Over the longer term, however, we anticipate that the limitations of a system that controls only the price of hospital care will become increasingly evident. There is simply too much discretion in hospitalization and in treatment of a hospitalized patient for price controls to serve as effective constraints on total hospital expenditures for the Medicare program. More comprehensive reforms such as hospital-based budgeting or prepaid care will likely rise to the top of policymakers' agendas. Indeed, when this occurs, we anticipate that the more comprehensive a reform, the more attractive it will seem. From this perspective, an all-payers system based on prospective budget targets has much to recommend it, controlling both volume and price and ensuring similar incentives for all purchasers of hospital care.

The DRGs may serve as a useful intermediate step in this process. The implementation and adjustments of Medicare's current PPS have taught us a great deal about the factors that affect the costs of hospital care. This information is useful, probably even necessary, to construct fair and effective capitation rates, hospital budgets and budget targets. Whichever direction the Medicare system takes—and it may move in several simultaneously—it can thus build on the lessons learned in the recent past and the near future.

NOTES

1. Considering all available evidence, one study concluded that the Professional Standards Review Organization (PSRO) program as a cost-control mechanism was slightly successful: "A small step in the right direction," with potential that remains to be tapped (Berman and Gertman, 1981, p. 60).

2. In practice, the Health Care Financing Administration (HCFA) has been extremely reticent to authorize outlier payments (Vladeck, 1985).

3. This attitude differs markedly from the approach taken by the Social Security Administration when Medicare was first implemented. Administrators went to extreme lengths to ensure that beneficiaries had access to the hospital located nearest their home (Feder, 1977).

4. Preliminary data indicates, however, that in the second half of 1984 and early 1985 length of stay remained almost constant (U.S. Congress, Office of Technology Assessment, 1985).

5. Much of this may reflect a concern over increased standardization of physician practices within the hospital (Arthur Anderson and Co., 1984).

6. Perhaps the most commonly proposed alternative to the prospective payment system (PPS) is capitation—paying a health maintenance organization (HMO) or some other prepaid plan a flat annual rate per patient for providing both ambulatory and hospital care. Prepayment offers some important advantages and some disadvantages compared to other methods of reimbursement. These are explored in Chapter 7. We do not expect, however, that prepayment represents a realistic alternative to PPS for all Medicare enrollees, at least in the near future. Even the most optimistic projections of enrollment in HMOs suggest that less than half the country will be enrolled in these organizations by the turn of the century (Schlesinger et al., 1986). It is important, therefore, to carefully consider options for improving Medicare's fee-for-service reimbursement system.

7. A similar evolution occurred in New Jersey's DRG system (Hsiao et al., 1986).

8. A similar rationale lies behind Medicare's special treatment of hospitals that are the sole provider in their community. If these hospitals were to specialize, beneficiaries might be forced to travel long distances to find care. To avoid creating large cost pressures on these facilities, professional-payment-system (PPS) reimbursement rates are based only partially on the national diagnostic-related-groups (DRG) rate; the institution's historical costs are the principal determinant of payment.

9. Public hospitals also must care for an increasing number of unprofitable patients who are dumped from private hospitals (Schiff et al., 1986). To the extent hospitals are able to distinguish patients who will be unprofitable to treat under DRGs it is likely that they will also be transferred or otherwise deposited in public hospitals.

10. Research indicates that hospitals located in all-payers states are less likely to discourage admission by Medicare recipients (Schlesinger et al., 1986).

11. New Jersey, for example, has an all-payers diagnostic-related-group system; Massachusetts administers an all-payers system based on budget targets for hospitals.

12. In the academic literature, the term "mixed reimbursement" is sometimes used synonomously with the term "blended reimbursement" (Ellis, 1986).

13. Though other states (e.g., Connecticut) have experienced large numbers of appeals as individual hospitals have sought special treatment.

14. Because hospital utilization across the country fell during this period, however, it is difficult to determine how much of these effects are due to the incentives of target budgets.

REFERENCES

American Hospital Association, Office of Public Policy Analysis. 1984. *Medicare PPS Equity Adjustments: An Analysis of Medicare/Low-Income Patient Involvement and other Hospital Factors*. Chicago: American Hospital Association.

Arthur Anderson and Co. 1984. *Health Care in the 1990s: Trends and Strategies*. Chicago.

Barnes, M. 1986. Discharge Procedure at Hospitals Criticized. *Boston Globe*, April 27:38.

Bentkover, J. D., F. A. Sloan, F. G. Feeley et al. 1984. Hospital Capital and Operating Costs. *Advances in Health Economics and Health Services Research* 5:213–36.

Berenson, R. A., and L. G. Pawlson. 1984. The Medicare Prospective Payment System and the Care of the Frail Elderly. *Journal of the American Geriatrics Society* 31 (11):843–84.

Berman, D. E., and P. M. Gertman. 1981. Cost Containment and Quality Assurance: The Potential and Performance of the Professional Standards Review Organization. In *Federal Health Programs*, ed. S. Altman and H. Sapolsky, pp. 43–61. Lexington, MA: Lexington Books.

Bonner, P. 1976. *On Site Utilization Review: An Evaluation of the Impact of Utilization Patterns and Expenditures* (Monograph), pp. 122–29. Boston: Harvard School of Public Health.

Brook, R. H., and K. N. Williams. 1976. Evaluation of the New Mexico Peer Review System: 1971–1973. *Medical Care* 14, Supplement.

Brown, E. 1983. Public Hospitals on the Brink: Their Problems and Their Options. *Journal of Health Politics, Policy and Law* 7 (4):927–44.

Carter, C. 1986. *Hospital Cost Containment in Massachusetts*. Ph.D. diss., MIT.

Chiswick, B. 1974. Hospital Utilization: An Analysis of SMSA Differences in Hospital Admission Rates, Occupancy Rates, and Bed Rates. National Bureau of Economic Research (NBER) Working Paper No. 2, May.

Dans, P., J. Weiner and S. Otter. 1985. Peer Review Organizations: Promises and Pitfalls. *New England Journal of Medicine* 313 (18):1131–37.

Davidson, S., J. Cromwell and R. Schurman. 1986. Medicaid Myths: Trends in Medicaid Expenditures and the Prospects of Reform. *Journal of Health Politics, Policy and Law* 10 (4):699–728.

Davis, K., and C. Schoen. 1978. *Health and the War on Poverty: A Ten-Year Appraisal.* Washington: Brookings Institution.

Davis, K., G. Anderson, S. Renn et al. 1985. Is Cost Containment Working? *Health Affairs* 4 (3):81–94.

Detsky, A. S., S. Stacey and C. Bombardier. 1983. The Effectiveness of a Regulatory Strategy in Containing Hospital Costs: The Ontario Experience, 1967–1981. *New England Journal of Medicine* 309 (3):151–59.

Dobson, A., J. G. Greer, R. H. Carlson et al. 1978. PSROs: Their Current Status and Their Impacts to Date. *Inquiry* 15 (Spring):113–28.

Eby, C., and D. R. Cohodes. 1985. What Do We Know About Rate-Setting? *Journal of Health Politics, Policy and Law* 10 (2):299–328.

Ellis, R. P. 1986. *Payment System for Addressing Systematic Risk in a Prospective Payment System.* Paper presented at the Research Issues in Economics and Mental Health Seminar. Sponsored by the National Institute of Mental Health, Andover, MA, June 19–20.

Ellis, R. P., and T. G. McGuire. 1986. Provider Behavior Under Prospective Reimbursement: Cost Sharing and Supply. *Journal of Health Economics* 5 (2):129–52.

Evans, Robert G. 1985. Illusions of Necessity: Evading Responsibility for Choice in Health Care. *Journal of Health Politics, Policy and Law* 10 (3):439–67.

Feder, J. M. 1977. *Medicare: The Politics of Federal Hospital Insurance.* Lexington, MA: D. C. Heath.

Feldstein, P. 1978. *Health Associations and the Demand for Legislation.* Cambridge, MA: Ballinger.

Gertman, P. M., and S. Lowenstein. 1984. A Research Paradigm for Severity Adjustment to Diagnosis-Related Groups. *Health Care Financing Review, 1984 Annual Supplement*, pp. 79–90.

Gertman, P., A. Monheit, J. Anderson et al. 1978. Utilization Review in the United States: Results from a 1976–1977 National Survey of Hospitals. *Medical Care* 17, Supplement.

Glenn, K., and J. Brazda. 1985a. DRGs and Quality of Care. *Perspectives* (January 7):1.

———. 1985b. Patient Dumping Mars Competitive Model. *Perspectives* (July 15):1.

———. 1985c. DRGs and Quality of Care. *Perspectives* (November 25):1.

Grimaldi, P. L. 1981. DRG Reimbursement in New Jersey: Some Initial Results. *Hospital Progress* (11):41–45.

Guterman, S., and A. Dobson. 1986. Impact of the Medicare Prospective Payment System for Hospitals. *Health Care Financing Review* 7 (3):97–114.

Harvey, L. 1986. *AMA Surveys of Physician and Public Opinion: 1986.* Chicago: American Medical Association.

Health Research and Educational Trust of New Jersey. 1984. *DRG Evaluation, Volume II, Economic and Financial Analysis.* Princeton, NJ.

Hellinger, F. J. 1976. The Effect of Certificate-of-Need Legislation on Hospital Investment. *Inquiry* 13 (Spring):187–93.

Horn, S. D., R. A. Horn and P. D. Sharkey. 1984. The Severity of Illness Index as a Severity Adjustment to Diagnosis-Related Groups. *Health Care Financing Review, 1984 Annual Supplement*, pp. 33–46.

Howell, J. 1981. *Regulating Hospital Capital Investment: The Experience in Massachusetts*, DHHS/Health Resources Administration, Pub. No. (DHS) 81–3298, March. Hyattsville, MD.

Hsiao, W. C., H. M. Sapolsky, D. L. Dunn et al. 1986. Lessons of the New Jersey DRG Payment System. *Health Affairs* 5 (2):32–45.

Iglehart, J. 1985. Medicare Turns to HMOs. *New England Journal of Medicine* 312 (2):132–37.

Ingaunzo, J., and M. Harju. 1985. What Makes Consumers Select a Hospital? Hospitals 59 (6):90–94.

Jencks, S. F., A. Dobson, P. Willis et al. 1984. Evaluating and Improving the Measurement of Hospital Case Mix. *Health Care Financing Review, 1984 Annual Supplement*, pp. 1–11.

Joskow, P. L. 1981. In *Controlling Hospital Costs: The Role of Government Regulation.* Cambridge, MA: MIT Press.

Kerschner, P. A. 1986. Are DRGs Affecting Just the Elderly? *Business Health* 3 (5):31–37.

Kuntz, E. 1984. Task Forces Scour Diagnosis, Therapy Methods for Cost-Cutting Procedures. *Modern Health Care* 14 (3):138–42.

Lave, J., and L. Lave. 1974. The Hospital Construction Act: An Evaluation of Hill-Burton Programs 1948–1973. Washington: American Enterprise Institute for Public Policy Research.

Lave, J., and S. Leinhardt. 1976. An Evaluation of a Hospital Stay Regulatory Mechanism. *American Journal of Public Health* 66 (8):959–67.

Law, S. 1974. *Blue Cross: What Went Wrong*. New Haven: Yale University Press.

Levenson, A. I. 1985. The For-Profit System. In *The New Economics and Psychiatric Care*, ed. S. S. Sharfstein and A. Beigel, 151–63. Washington: American Psychiatric Press.

Macro Systems, Inc. 1975. *The Certificate of Need Experiences: An Early Assessment.* Volume I, *Summary Report* No. NTIS HRP–1000190; Volume II, *State Reports* No. NTIS HRP–1000189. Springfield, VA: U.S. Department of Commerce, National Technical Information Service.

Marmor, T. R., M. Schlesinger, R. W. Smithey. 1986. A New Look at Nonprofits: Health Care Policy in a Competitive Age. *Yale Journal on Regulation* 3 (2):313–349.

May, J. J. 1975. Utilization of Health Services and the Availability of Resources. In *Equity in Health Services: Empirical Analyses in Social Policy*, ed. R. Anderson, J. Kravits and O. Anderson, 131–50. Cambridge, MA: Ballinger.

May, J. J., and J. Wasserman. 1984. Selected Results from an Evaluation of the New Jersey Diagnosis-Related Group System. *Health Service Research* 19 (5):547–59.

Meyer, J. A. 1986. Financing Uncompensated Care with All-Payer Rate Regulation. In *Uncompensated Hospital Care: Rights and Responsibilities*, ed. F. A. Sloan, J. F. Blumstein and J. M. Perrin, 167–84. Baltimore: Johns Hopkins University Press.

Mitchell, J. H., J. M. Hardacre, F. J. Wenzel et al. 1975. Cholecystectomy Peer Review: Measurement of Four Variables. *Medical Care* 13 (4):409–416.

Newcomer, R., J. Wood and A. Sankar. 1985. Medicare Prospective Payment: Anticipated Effect on Hospitals, Other Community Agencies, and Families. *Journal of Health Politics, Policy and Law* 10 (2):275–82.

Newhouse, J., and C. Phelps. 1976. New Estimates of Price and Income Elasticities of Medicare Services. In *The Role of Health Insurance in the Health Services Sector*, ed. R. Rossett, 216–313. New York: National Bureau of Economic Research.

Packer, C. L. 1985. Automation in the Medical Records Department. *Hospitals* 59 (5):100–104.

Pauly, M. V. 1986. Taxation, Health Insurance, and Market Failure in the Medical Economy. *Journal of Economic Literature* 24 (2):629–75.

Policy Analysis, Inc., and Urban Systems Research and Engineering, Inc. 1981. *Evaluation of the Effects of Certificate-of-Need Programs.* Sponsored by DHHS, Health Resources Administration, Contract No. 231–77–0114.

Porter, S. 1984. How Ohio Hospitals Are Coping with DRGs. *Ohio State Medical Journal* 80 (4):263–65.

Rice, T., G. de Lissovoy, J. Gabel et al. 1985. The State of PPOs: Results from a National Survey. *Health Affairs* 4(4):25–40.

Roemer, M. 1961. Bed Supply and Hospitalization: Natural Equipment. *Hospitals* 34:35–42.
———. 1976. Hospital Utilization and the Health Care System. *American Journal of Public Health* 66 (8):953–954.
Rosko, M. D., and R. W. Broyles. 1986. The Impact of the New Jersey All-Payer DRG System. *Inquiry* 23 (1):67–75.
Rothenberg, E. 1976. *Regulation and Expansion of Health Facilities: The Certificate of Need Experience in New York State*. New York: Praeger.
Rowe, J. W. 1985. Health Care of the Elderly. *New England Journal of Medicine* 312 (13):827–35.
Schiff, R., D. Ansell, J. Schlosser et al. 1986. Transfers to a Public Hospital: A Prospective Study of 467 Patients. *New England Journal of Medicine* 314 (9):552–57.
Schlesinger, M. 1985. The Rise of Proprietary Health Care. *Business and Health* 2 (1):7–12.
Schlesinger, M., T. Wetle and J. H. Morse. 1984. Improving Care of the Older Veteran: Issues and Options. In *Older Veterans: Linking VA and Community Resources*, ed. T. Wetle and J. W. Rowe, 409–33. Cambridge: Harvard University Press.
Schlesinger, M., J. Bentkover, D. Blumenthal et al. 1986. Multihospital Systems and Access to Health Care. In *Advances in Health Economics and Health Services Research*, Volume 7, ed. L. Rossiter, R. Scheffler, G. Wilensky et al. Greenwich, CT: JAI Press.
Schweiker, R. S. 1982. Report to Congress on Hospital Prospective Payment for Medicare.
Siegel, C., E. Laska and S. Lin. 1986. *Decision Theory Models for Payment Schemes. A Negotiated Approach Between Payers and Providers*. Paper presented at the Research Issues in Economics and Mental Health Seminar. Sponsored by the National Institute of Mental Health, Andover, MA, June 19–20.
Sigmond, R. M. 1985. *Re-Examining the Role of the Community Hospital in a Competitive Environment*. The 1985 Michael M. Davis Lecture. Millwood, VA: Project HOPE.
Sloan, F. A. 1983. Rate Regulation as a Strategy for Hospital Cost Control: Evidence from the Last Decade. *Milbank Memorial Fund Quarterly* 61(2):195–221.
Sloan, F. A., and B. Steinwald. 1980. Effects of Regulation on Hospital Costs and Input Use. *Journal of Law and Economics* 23 (1):81–110.
Starr, P. 1982. *The Social Transformation of American Medicine*. New York: Basic Books.
Sullivan, R. 1985. Decline in Hospital Use Tied to New U.S. Policies. *New York Times* April 16:1.
Taube, C. A., E. S. Lee and R. N. Forthofer. 1984. DRGs in Psychiatry: An Empirical Evaluation. *Medical Care* 22(7):597–610.
Thompson, F. J. 1981. *Health Policy and the Bureaucracy: Politics and Implementation*. Cambridge: MIT Press.
U.S. Congress. Office of Technology Assessment. 1985. *Medicare's Prospective Payment System: Strategies for Evaluating Cost, Quality, and Medical Technology*. OTA-H-262.
U.S. Congressional Budget Office. 1980. *The Impact of PSROs on Health Care Costs: 1980 Update of the CBO Evaluation*. Staff Draft Analysis, May 2.
U.S. Department of Health and Human Services. National Center for Health Statistics, Public Health Service. 1984. *Health, United States 1984*. DHHS Pub. No. (PHS85-1232.
U.S. General Accounting Office. 1987. *Discharge Planners Report Increasing Difficulty in Placing Medicare Patients*. Pub. No. GAO/OPEMD-87-5BR.
Vaida, M. 1984. The Financial Impact of Prospective Payment on Hospitals. *Health Affairs* 3 (1):112–19.
Vladeck, B. C. 1985. Reforming Medicare Provider Payment. *Journal of Health Politics, Policy and Law* 10 (3):513–32.
Wennberg, J. E., K. McPherson and P. Caper. 1984. Will Payment Based on Diagnosis-Related Groups Control Hospital Costs? *New England Journal of Medicine* 311 (5):295–300.

Wilensky, G. R. 1986. Underwriting Uninsured: Targeting Providers or Individuals. In *Uncompensated Hospital Care: Rights and Responsibilities*, ed. F. A. Sloan, J. F. Blumstein and J. M. Perrin, 148–66. Baltimore: Johns Hopkins University Press.

Worthington, N. L., and P. A. Piro. 1982. The Effects of Hospital Rate-Setting Programs on Volumes of Hospital Services: A Preliminary Analysis. *Health Care Financing Review* 4 (2):47–61.

6

Payment of Physicians Under Medicare

David Blumenthal
William Hsiao

After the extensive recent reforms in methods of paying for hospital care under Part A of Medicare (discussed in detail in Chapter 5), attention has shifted to payments to physicians under Part B of the program. Part B is an optional supplementary medical insurance (SMI) program that covers part of the cost of physician services and other outpatient and noninstitutional services, including some laboratory tests. To be insured under SMI, elderly citizens must pay a monthly premium, which, in 1987 was $17.90. These premium payments pay for about 25 percent of SMI expenditures for the elderly. The balance is financed out of general federal revenues through a congressional appropriation. Just over 97 percent of the elderly now opt to purchase SMI coverage.

Payments to physicians account for about 75 percent of expenditures under Medicare Part B (U.S. Congress, Office of Technology Assessment, 1986). When it enacted a prospective payment system (PPS) for hospitals, Congress directed the secretary of Health and Human Services to report back by the end of 1985 with recommendations for reform. This directive reflected widespread concern about problems with physician services available to Medicare patients and about the ways in which payment methods affect those difficulties. However, as of this writing, the secretary has not forwarded to the Congress official proposals for changing the way physicians are paid under Medicare.

Perhaps anticipating these delays in instituting comprehensive physician payment reform, Congress in 1986 created the Physician Payment Review Commission. This 13-member group is charged with reviewing current methods of compensating physicians and advising Congress on how those methods should be reformed (Physician Payment Review Commission, 1987).

Problems: Physicians' Services

As in the Medicare program generally, the physician component of the program (Medicare Part B) faces at least two basic problems: high costs and persistent inequities in its treatment of physicians and patients.

High Costs

The costs of physician services under Medicare are large and increasing rapidly. In 1986, Medicare spent $19.2 billion for physicians' services, up from $4 billion in 1976 (Pear, 1987). Expenditures for physician services are growing more rapidly than any other component of Medicare or any other program in the federal domestic budget. Over the 10 years from 1975–84, Medicare payments to physicians grew at an average annual rate of 18.5 percent. Over the period 1979–84, these expenditures grew 21 percent yearly (U.S. Congress, Senate, 1984). In contrast, Medicare's expenditures for hospital services grew by 15.7 percent annually over the 5 years prior to 1984. In the 1983–1986 period, Medicare spending on physicians' services grew at an annual rate of 9.1 percent, compared to 8.2 percent for hospitals (Anderson and Erickson, 1987). Since 1978, Medicare's expenditures per beneficiary on physicians' services have generally exceeded per capita expenditures on physicians' services for the nation as a whole (U.S. Congress, Office of Technology Assessment, 1986).

The increases in Medicare's payments to physicians have resulted from several factors. Over the period 1975–82, general inflation (measured by increases in the consumer price index [CPI]) accounted for about 40 percent of the growth in physician reimbursement, whereas increases in Medicare enrollment—reflecting the aging of the population—accounted for another 13 percent. These factors are largely beyond the control of either policymakers or physicians.

An additional 34 percent of the increase in payments to physicians, however, resulted from greater intensity of services—the delivery of more services per enrollee and the increasing complexity of services. A further 12 percent reflected real increases in physician charges—that is, increases greater than the rate of inflation (Juba, 1985). These last two factors—increases in the intensity of services provided and in the fees physicians charge—seem more susceptible than general inflation or increasing Medicare enrollment to cost control measures. They, therefore, deserve special scrutiny.

Real Increases in Fees

One of the most important factors behind the rise in the fees that physicians charge Medicare has been the way the program pays physicians. A description of how the system works follows.

After physicians see Medicare patients, the physicians must first decide whether to accept assignment for the services they provide. By accepting assignment, physicians allow patients to assign to them the right to bill Medicare directly for the service or services they have rendered. This relieves patients of the paperwork involved in getting paid by Medicare and assures the physicians that they will be promptly and reliably reimbursed. (Physicians can decide whether to accept assignment on a service-by-service [bill-by-bill] basis.) If they have to wait for patients to get paid by Medicare before collecting, physicians may have to wait longer; even then, patients could conceivably refuse to turn the full Medicare payment over to physicians.

Though accepting assignment has advantages for physicians, it also has one major disadvantage: Physicians who bill Medicare directly must agree to accept

Medicare's "reasonable charge" as payment in full. Medicare's reasonable charge is, in turn, established according to the "customary, prevailing and reasonable" (CPR) methodology. Specifically, for each service that a physician bills Medicare, that program pays the lowest of the following amounts: (1) the amount of the physician's actual bill for the service, (2) the amount the physician customarily charges the majority of his patients for the service (i.e, the amount the physician charges most of the time), or (3) the prevailing charge for the service, which is set by law at the 75th percentile of the customary charges of all physicians within a given medical specialty within the area. Thus, whichever of these three amounts is lowest is the "reasonable charge" for that service for Medicare purposes. Medicare itself will pay only 80 percent of this amount and will only pay that much once the patient has exhausted his or her deductible under Part B for the year in question. For the portion Medicare will not pay, the physician is allowed to bill the patient directly.

When physicians decline assignment, they are then free to bill patients any amount they please for the services they delivered. This allows them to collect more than Medicare allows and assures them that Medicare will not be able to tightly control their fees or income from elderly patients. The catch, of course, is that they must collect directly from the patients. Patients, in turn, can then submit the physician's bill directly to Medicare. Under these circumstances, Medicare will pay the patient what they would have paid the physician: the "reasonable charge" minus appropriate coinsurance and deductibles.

Actually, the federal government itself only rarely gets involved in these transactions because it generally contracts with private insurance companies to administer the system and handle the bills and payments. These insurance companies are called Medicare carriers. One of the most common carriers is Blue Shield. Though they operate under federal guidelines and supervision, carriers have considerable discretion in determining the amount physicians should be paid. They also determine what an area or locality should consist of for the purpose of determining prevailing fees. Generally, these areas consist of economic or political subdivisions of states.

This system is obviously very complex (a drawback in itself because it is not only costly to administer but also confusing for both patients and physicians alike). One of its most problematic features, however, is its inherent tendency to push up physicians' fees. Under the CPR methodology, physicians have an incentive to increase the amount they bill Medicare for a given service. By doing so, they increase their profile of customary charges (what Medicare records as the amount they usually bill patients), thus potentially raising the amount Medicare will pay them. Increases in individual physicians' customary charges also lead to increases in the prevailing charge for the area, thus making it possible for all physicians to receive higher payments.

The inflationary tendency of the CPR methodology partly accounts for the real increase in physicians' fees under Medicare. Another factor, however, has been the tendency for physicians' charges to remain high even when costs go down. When introduced, new procedures (such as coronary bypass surgery or endoscopy) have tended to be reimbursed generously because they required considerable time and knowledge on the part of pioneering physicians. Once such procedures become routine, however, the CPR methodology has no mechanism for reducing physicians' fees unless doctors themselves lower the amounts for which they bill patients.

Increases in Intensity of Service

Between 1975 and 1982, the number of physicians' services used by the average Medicare beneficiary increased by 6 percent per year. Utilization of specialists' services, which tend to be more complex and costly, increased faster than services provided by generalists (Juba, 1985). This growing intensity of physicians' services has roots both in the methods Medicare uses to pay doctors and in broader currents in the medical care system such as in the increasing supply of physicians. Medicare's payment methods contribute to the use of more services and more complex services in several ways.

First, Medicare pays physicians on a fee-for-service basis; a physician is generally entitled to a separate payment from the program for every service provided—such as an office visit or a surgical procedure. This encourages physicians to provide more services. It is widely recognized that, within limits, physicians play an important role in deciding how often patients visit them and what services they receive; this is especially true for patients with chronic illnesses, which are particularly common among the elderly (Wilensky and Rossiter, 1983). Second, the CPR methodology has tended to maintain historic disparities in the fees charged by physicians. For instance, specialists and surgeons, traditionally paid more for their services, have tended to do better under Medicare than primary care practitioners.[1] Specialists, in particular, usually have a costly style of practice. They tend to order more tests and more complicated tests than primary physicians. Surgeons, similarly, provide expensive treatment. In undergoing surgery, patients also generally require consultant services, laboratory tests and many other services covered by Medicare Parts A and B. By paying specialists and surgeons more, Medicare encourages them to provide more of these costly services and simultaneously increases their income, thus encouraging young physicians to enter those fields and exacerbating the current excess supply of specialists and surgeons.

A number of factors not attributable to Medicare also underlie the increasing use and complexity of physicians' services. The growing supply of physicians is perhaps most important. Between 1960 and 1980, the number of physicians per 100,000 citizens in this country increased by 21 percent, from 156 to 197. By the year 2000, the number is expected to grow an additional 19 percent, to 233 per 100,000. The number of specialists is growing faster than the number of primary care practitioners (Tarlov, 1986).

Many analysts believe that the growth in the supply of physicians has exceeded growth in demand and that to maintain their incomes, some physicians have encouraged the use of more health care services than necessary. Although in a normal competitive market such an increase in the supply of services would be expected to depress prices, the medical marketplace has not behaved this way. One reason is that the availability of insurance has protected consumers from the cost of services; thus consumers have not shopped around for physicians with the lowest prices. The competitive dynamic, therefore, has never taken hold, and prices have actually increased.

The availability of new, more expensive health care technologies has also undoubtedly played a role in increasing the complexity and costliness of physicians' services. It is a reflection of the changing nature of medicine during Medicare's brief lifetime that the number of items listed in the American Medical Association's (AMA's) current procedure codes (which define services for billing purposes) tripled between 1966 and 1978 (U.S. Congress, Senate, 1984).

Inequities

The way in which Medicare pays physicians also promotes inequitable treatment of different physician and patient groups. The payment system's effect on patients is discussed extensively in Chapter 3, but several points deserve reiteration.

Medicare imposes very different cost burdens on different groups of eligible patients. Out-of-pocket expenditures for health care represent 17 percent of net income for low-income elders but only 1.4 percent of income for those with high income (see Table 3–2). Out-of-pocket expenditures are 40 percent higher among Medicare patients in the Western region of the U.S. than among those in the North Central region.

Two features of Medicare's method of reimbursing physicians contribute to such income-related and geographic inequities. First, physicians do not receive the full "reasonable charge" when they bill Medicare. Patients are responsible for paying coinsurance (generally 20 percent of the Medicare allowed fee) and the deductible ($75 in 1987). Because these payments are not adjusted for income, they fall more heavily on patients with lower incomes.

Second, when physicians refuse assignment and bill in excess of Medicare's reasonable charge, patients have to make up the difference. Consequently, they may be subject to substantial and often unpredictable out-of-pocket expenses as well as additional paperwork requirements (because they must bill Medicare themselves to collect what they are owed). In 1982, physicians accepted assignment for about 53 percent of the claims submitted to Medicare (U.S. Congress, Senate, 1984). In the 47 percent of cases where physicians billed patients directly, their bills exceeded what Medicare would pay 86 percent of the time. The average excess amount was $28.10 (U.S. Congress, Senate, 1983). Once again, these costs fall more heavily on the poor than on the well-to-do.

The rate at which physicians accept assignment has been increasing gradually in recent years, reaching 59 percent of claims in 1984, 69 percent in 1985, and 74.1 percent in 1987 (U.S. Congress, Office of Technology Assessment, 1986; Gornick et al., 1985; Medicine & Health, 1987). The large jump in physicians accepting assignment resulted in part from a new program introduced in 1984 that promised physicians who accepted assignment on all cases (so-called participating physicians) that they would receive greater increases in their fees than nonparticipating doctors.

The way Medicare pays physicians creates inequities among doctors. Medicare rates favor specialists over primary care physicians. In 1982, for example, specialists were paid 20 to 53 percent more for office visits than were primary care physicians (U.S. Congress, Senate, 1984). The CPR method also leads to considerable disparities in rates of reimbursement for comparable services among different geographic areas. In 1980, Medicare's prevailing fees for a brief follow-up visit by an internist ranged from $7.00 in certain areas of Wisconsin to $33.10 in New York City (U.S. Congress, Office of Technology Assessment, 1986). In many cases, these different payment rates have no clear justification. They are not based on the intrinsic value of the services performed or the cost of performing them. But they do affect the income of physicians, their choice of specialty, the rates at which they peform procedures and the availability of care in different areas. The higher rates paid doctors in urban areas, for example, help to explain why there are fewer physicians in rural areas.

Thus, Medicare payment rates not only discriminate unfairly against certain groups of physicians, but exert perverse effects on access to, and cost of, care for Medicare beneficiaries. Under any payment scheme, differences in rates of payment among physicians would be inevitable. However, there is a widespread feeling that these variations should reflect legitimate differences in the value attached to services or the cost of providing them rather than merely the customary and prevailing charge levels in communities.

Past Efforts at Reform

The problems created by Medicare's payment method have been apparent to policymakers for some time, and several previous efforts have been made to improve reimbursement policy. In 1972, responding to dramatic increases in physicians' charges between 1966 and 1971, Congress enacted the current rule that Medicare will pay no more for a service than the 75th percentile of the customary charges of all physicians in the area for that service (rather than the 95th percentile, that had previously been the rule). In addition, Congress stipulated that the payment for a particular service in a given region could not rise faster than an economic index reflecting earning levels and physicians' operating expenses. In 1980, Congress limited the amount physicians could bill for laboratory services performed in their offices. Nevertheless, Medicare payments to physicians continued to rise rapidly.

In 1984, responding to the continued escalation of physicians' fees and program costs, Congress froze physician payments at 1984 levels until May 1, 1986 for "participating physicians" (those accepting assignment for all cases), and until January 1, 1987 for other doctors (Physician Payment Review Commission, 1987). Since the lifting of the fee freeze, HCFA has limited the amount that non-participating physicians can increase their charges, but has not done so for participating physicians (Physician Payment Review Commission, 1987).

In 1985 and 1986, Congress took further steps to control costs of physicians' services by requiring that physicians' fees under Medicare meet a test of "inherent reasonableness." Under criteria set forth by the Congress, charges for a particular service in a particular locality might be considered unreasonable if they were significantly above or below charges for the same service in other localities (after taking into account differences in physicians' costs in different areas). Similarly, a particular physicians' charges might fail the inherent reasonableness test if his or her fees were significantly higher or lower than other physicians' charges for the same service in the same locality (Physician Payment Review Commission, 1987). As a first application of the inherent reasonableness test, Congress required that allowed charges for cataract surgery and related anesthesia be reduced by 10 percent in 1987, and a further 2 percent in 1988.

Unfortunately, there is little evidence that recent controls on physicians' fees have proven more successful in controlling Medicare expenditures than earlier reforms. During fiscal year 1986, Medicare physician expenditures increased by 11.1

percent, 11 times faster than the rate of increase in the CPI (Anderson and Erickson, 1987).

The primary reason for this continued escalation of overall costs is that neither the freeze on physicians' fees nor any of the previous reforms addressed the fundamental problems created by Medicare's payment methods. Specifically, none of the cost-containment efforts undertaken to date has reduced the ability of physicians to increase the number of services for which they can bill Medicare. Physicians can either recommend more care for their patients or unbundle services—that is, break up the care they provide into a larger number of billable units (Rice and McCall, 1982; Rice, 1983). For example, instead of including certain routine laboratory tests in the cost of an office visit, physicians can bill separately for the tests, generating more income in the process. It is notable, for example, that though the number of physician visits used each year by the average beneficiary has stayed relatively stable since Medicare was enacted, the number of claims filed per beneficiary under Part B has increased more than sevenfold (U.S. Congress, Office of Technology Assessment, 1986).

Freezes on fees also leave untouched existing disparities in the rates at which different groups of physicians are paid. Moreover, they do little or nothing to address inequities in the cost burden borne by Medicare patients; freezes may even increase existing inequities if more physicians refuse assignment in the hope of receiving from patients what they cannot get from Medicare.

Options for Reform

Any physician payment system proposed for Medicare must answer three basic questions:

- On what unit of care should payment be based?
- What should the rates of payment be, and how should they be set?
- How, if at all, should Medicare encourage or require that physicians accept Medicare's rate as payment in full?

The answers to these questions affect our critical concerns: How much physicians are paid, the quality of care they provide and how equitably Medicare treats physicians, patients and other participants in the health care system.

The unit of care for which Medicare pays can take any of three forms. Medicare can continue to pay for each individual service actually provided (fee-for-service care or piecework), the program can pay a set amount for each episode of illness (as Medicare now does for hospital care under Medicare Part A), or it can pay a lump sum for all the care to be received by an enrollee during a year or some other defined period (capitation).

Once the unit of payment is determined, the amount Medicare will pay for each service, illness or period of care must be established. Again, there are several possibilities. Medicare could pay physicians based on the going rate for that type of care—that is, the amount that they have historically or customarily charged other patients for the same type of care. This is what the CPR methodology has done for fee-for-service care, though Congress has now limited the rate of inflation for those fees. Or the government can step in and decide itself (in consultation with experts and providers) what a given type of service is worth using some standard of value, either relative to other services or absolutely. These two methods are not mutually exclusive. Historical rates of payment may provide a guide to the value of services in certain circumstances.

Whatever units and rates of payment are chosen, Medicare must also deal with the question of whether doctors should be limited to the rates set by the program. Under the present system, physicians are permitted to charge patients the "unassigned" portion of their ordinary fees—that is, the amount beyond the "reasonable charge" set by Medicare. This increases the aggregate cost of health care, but it makes physicians more willing to accept Medicare patients.

These are the primary issues that we will now be considering as we describe and evaluate several proposals for improving the ways Medicare pays physicians. What follows is by no means a comprehensive list of options, and details could vary. The choices presented are intended to illustrate the major directions for reform and the advantages and disadvantages of each. It should be noted that each of the reforms discussed here is currently under active consideration by policymakers.

In thinking about ways to reform physician payment, it is useful to keep in mind one further factor in the success or failure of any reform: The reaction of physicians to changes in payment methods and thus to potential limitations on their income and style of practice. Although some aspects of Medicare's current policy may seem irrational in hindsight, they often represent past responses to concerns about the acceptability of the program to physicians; these concerns remain relevant today.

The generosity of the CPR method and the flexibility allowed physicians in accepting or rejecting assignment, for instance, were intended to mitigate opposition to the enactment of Medicare in 1965 and to encourage physicians to participate in the program. Even today, more than twenty years after Medicare was established, attempts to change its payment policy must still contend with political opposition from physicians' groups such as the AMA, which will amost certainly oppose restrictions on physicians' freedom to set and collect their own fees. In contrast, the hospital industry generally supported the changes in hospital reimbursement passed in 1983.

Widespread discontent on the part of physicians with any reforms in payment methods could restrict access to care for Medicare beneficiaries because some physicians might choose to see fewer Medicare patients or none at all.[2] Even relatively minor changes in payment policy could encourage such changes in behavior. Revolutionary changes such as the sudden institution of a prepaid system for most patients (e.g., the one now in place in Great Britain) could conceivably cause mass defections from the program. One study showed that if physicians were required to take all Medicare patients on assignment or not take any patients on assignment, only 20 percent of internists would opt for assignment (Mitchell and Cromwell, 1983). This would result in fewer Medicare patients seeing internists on an assigned basis and an increase in the cost of care for many elderly individuals. Internists are the chief providers of primary care for elderly patients.

One apparently simple deterrent to physician noncooperation with the Medicare program would be to require as a condition of licensure that they treat Medicare patients at a price determined by the government. Massachusetts has recently adopted legislation requiring physicians to do this, and the Supreme Court has upheld the law's constitutionality. However, even if this policy were desirable, it seems politically untenable at the national level during the time period with which we are concerned.

In reviewing options for changes in payment to physicians, policymakers should also keep in mind the differences between physicians and hospitals as providers of health care. Despite the apparent success of recent measures to contain hospital costs, the prospective methods used for paying hospitals may not be appropriate for paying physicians. One important difference between physicians and hospitals, for instance, is the physician's traditional role as the agent of the patient. Physicians make most of the decisions that affect the nature of treatment and the quality of patient care. Their ability and willingness to advocate patients' interests is, therefore, critical to patient well-being and peace of mind. This is particularly true now that payment is based on diagnostic-related groups (DRG) under Part A. This has given hospitals the incentive to discharge patients as early as possible and provide fewer services, thus creating fears that Medicare patients will be discharged "sicker and quicker" (see Chapter 5).

A second difference between physicians and hospitals is that physicians, especially those in small groups or solo practices, are less able than hospitals to bear the financial risks that are entailed in prospective payment schemes based either on an episode of illness or on a period of time. Hospitals care for many more Medicare patients than do physicians in a given year.[3] Thus, if hospitals lose a lot of money on a particular patient—for example, during a particular hospitalization—they are more likely to be able to make it up either through small gains on many patients or large gains on a few. Nonprofit hospitals also have the option of seeking charitable contributions to help cover deficits. Individual physicians do not have these options or the financial reserves to tolerate a string of bad luck.

Finally, despite their high incomes, and some signs of public disaffection (especially in the form of skyrocketing malpractice awards), physicians retain substantial popular respect and support in this country. The public may be more likely to support a payment system that inflicts financial hardship or even closure on some hospitals than one that causes severe financial difficulties for any appreciable number of physicians.

Physicians do not deserve a veto over proposed reforms. The interests of Medicare patients and the public at large should remain paramount in designing programs for paying physicians, and physician opposition to reasonable reforms should be expected and confronted head on. Nevertheless, any attempts to reform physician payment under Medicare must take account of physician reaction if the reforms are to enjoy enduring success.

Fee Schedules Based on a Relative Value Scale

One of the most widely discussed options for reforming physician payment proposes that Medicare continue to pay physicians on a fee-for-service basis but that government should set those fees itself instead of allowing physicians to set them as under the CPR methodology. The result would be a schedule of fees that would determine how much a physician could be paid for every recognized service.

A critical question, of course, is how exactly the Medicare program should calculate physician fees under a fee schedule. For example, how should the compensation for an office visit compare with the compensation for performing surgery? And how should the fee for a hernia operation compare with that for a heart transplant? As we have seen, a number of approaches are possible. Medicare could, for example, simply take existing fees as a guide but limit their growth rate much more aggressively than it has in the past. By freezing physicians' fees over the last two years, Medicare has already moved much closer to a de facto fee schedule of this type.

However, proponents of fee schedules generally advocate a more aggressive approach. They say that the Medicare program (in consultation with experts, physicians and other interested parties) should determine fees based on the relative values of each service. Taking into account the complexity of the physician service in question and the time and skill required to provide it, the government should assign each type of service a weight, or value, measured in relative value units (RVUs). An initial office visit, for instance, might be assigned 2.0 RVUs, a brief follow-up 1.0, and an appendectomy 6.5.

Once the intrinsic worth of a service were determined, the government would then have to decide how much to pay each physician in dollars and cents for performing it. The government would want to take into account issues of fairness and public policy. Physicians practicing in different geographic areas, for example, face different costs of living that affect their office expenses and the buying power of their after-tax income. Fairness requires that these variations in cost of living be factored into any compensation scheme. Similarly, the federal government may want to encourage physicians to live in certain underserved areas and to enter certain undersupplied specialties. One way to take these issues into account would be to develop a multiplier that would be higher or lower depending on a number of factors related to geography and specialty. The product of the relative value assigned a given service and an individual physician's multiplier would produce the final fee in dollars and cents.

Adopting a fee schedule of this type could contribute to controlling Medicare costs. The inflationary tendency built into the current CPR methodology would be reversed at a single stroke because the government, not physicians, would be setting fees. The Medicare program could also correct incentives in the current system that encourage the delivery of high-technology services when other, less costly services might suffice. For example, it could make certain that primary and preventive services are reimbursed more generously and specialty and surgical care less generously than is currently the case. Finally, the downward stickiness of physician fees could be overcome by reducing the number of RVUs assigned to services after they become routinized.

A fee schedule based on relative values has other advantages as well. It would partially rectify inequities in the way physicians are paid by Medicare. Although compensation would still vary by geography and specialty, the factors influencing those disparities would be out in the open, subject to discussion and negotiation, and presumably, related to the real costs of providing the service itself. Depending on how the issue of assignment were handled (see later discussion), the development and publication of a fee schedule might also make reimbursement more predictable for both physicians and patients. Patients, in particular, would be less likely to find themselves with large unexpected liabilities in the form of copayments for assigned claims.

Fee schedules also have disadvantages, though most of these can be partially rectified. One major weakness of this approach is that fee-for-service payment continues to encourage doctors to deliver more services in order to increase their incomes. This loophole could jeopardize its ability to control costs.

There are two possible solutions to this problem. First, the federal government could set an annual target level for physician expenditures and reduce multipliers across the board during the course of the year if it appeared that payments were likely to exceed that target. Second, Medicare could reduce the number of different services for which physicians bill the program from the current 7,500 to about 1,000. This would limit physicians' ability to unbundle services—that is, to break down a given service into many components for which separate bills could be submitted. Physicians have used this device in the past to increase their incomes in the face of restraints on Medicare fees.

Another problem with this approach to paying physicians is its complexity. Redefining and reducing the services for which physicians bill, developing a defensible RVU scale, calculating multipliers and adjusting all these program elements for changes in medical technology, standards of practice and trends in physician expenditures constitute a prodigious set of tasks. To deal with these challenges, it would be essential to phase in a fee schedule over a number of years. Also, the technical tasks could be delegated to a national commission on physician payment that would include health services researchers, economists, policymakers and physicians who, under instructions from federal officials, could be responsible for calculating RVUs for services and multipliers.

The inclusion of physicians and (perhaps) representatives of organized medicine on such a national commission might partially address another drawback of a fee schedule: the prospect of physician opposition. If physicians conclude that Medicare's payment rates offer inadequate compensation for certain services or if they feel those rates are arbitrary and unfair, they may simply stop providing such services to Medicare patients. But threats to access to care for Medicare patients may be minimized by seeking the input of physician representatives. Indeed, a number of physician groups, including the American College of Physicians (representing internists), the American College of Surgeons, and the AMA itself have begun intensive reviews of the fee-schedule option. The AMA is cooperating in a government-funded study of this approach (Medicine & Health, 1987). Among all the options available for reforming physician payment, this seems likely to be the most acceptable to American physicians. The reason may be that it preserves the fee-for-service approach to compensation and thus involves the least radical departure from current reimbursement methods.

Though not without its problems, the type of fee schedule outlined here would contribute to cost control and rectify some inequities in the current CPR methodology. It seems likely to be acceptable to physicians and could probably be implemented with a suitable phase-in period. On the whole, therefore, it would be an improvement over the current Medicare payment system. The question, however, is whether it is the best available alternative.

Lump-sum Payments for Episodes of Illness

Medicare now pays hospitals a single fee based on the patient's diagnosis for all care rendered a Medicare beneficiary during a hospital stay. This payment method is known informally as reimbusement by DRGs.

Some health policy analysts have recommended that Medicare pay physicians the same way: with a single payment based on the patient's diagnosis for all services provided a beneficiary during a complete episode of illness. Medicare could classify patients for reimbursement purposes using the same DRGs now used for hospital care (thus creating physician DRGs or MDDRGs) or it could create a new diagnostic classification scheme.

The basic advantage of this proposal is that Medicare's payment for each episode of illness would be set in advance; thus physicians could not increase their revenues by providing additional services or performing additional procedures. Paying by episode of illness directly combats one of the problems of a fee schedule: the opportunity and incentive for physicians to dispense more care. Allowing physicians to retain some of the savings might even stimulate them to find new, more cost-effective approaches to caring for patients with a given illness. The adoption of PPS for hospital care in 1983 is partly responsible for slowing the growth in Medicare's expenditures for hospital services.

There are, however, several disadvantages to paying physicians by episode of illness. Most important is concern about its effect on quality of patient care. Reimbursement on the basis of MDDRGs or some similar scheme creates incentives for physicians to reduce the quantity of services they provide patients. Because physicians would not receive any additional revenue from, for example, visiting hospitalized patients, they might be tempted to eliminate some visits and use their time in other ways. To the extent physicians have provided unneeded services or provided needed services inefficiently, this result may be desirable from the standpoint of cost containment. The question, however, is whether, knowingly or unknowingly, physicians will also skimp on essential care. If this occurred, the sickest patients in any diagnostic category would be placed in the greatest jeopardy. Their care would be more time-consuming than average, but the physician would be paid only the average fee.

Paying physicians by episode of illness, therefore, may tend to jeopardize the physician's willingness to act as the patient's advocate. It would also directly align physicians' financial incentives with those of hospitals. Both would benefit from providing fewer services and discharging patients more quickly. The quality of hospital care, therefore, might be particularly susceptible to manipulation.

Other problems confront this approach to reimbursing physicians. A patient may receive care from several physicians during an episode of illness, some within the hospital, others outside it. Proponents of using the episode of illness as a unit of payment, however, envision a lump sum intended to pay for all physicians' services the beneficiary receives. As a result, some method must be developed of distributing the Medicare payment among all the physicians who treat each patient. For hospital care alone it may be possible to require that physicians on the hospital staff organize themselves into a group that would receive and distribute the payment. The hospital itself might also receive the reimbursement, acting as agent for the physicians who are affiliated with it. But what about situations in which physicians from another hospital or physicians without hospital privileges are involved? A number of such technical issues have not been addressed as yet.

Another difficulty concerns the definition of episode of illness. For inpatient care the period of the hospital stay, possibly along with certain follow-up care, can serve as a reasonable definition of episode of illness. However, the limits are not so clear for conditions handled on an outpatient basis. Before physicians can be reimbursed for taking a patient through a particular illness, much more work will be required to develop standard definitions of the beginning and end of such events, and then to decide how much each such event is worth.

In defining episodes of illness and the resource cost of caring for them, it will be essential to take diagnosis into account. Obviously, caring for an ulcer on an outpatient basis may require different amounts of physician time and laboratory tests than caring for an episode of the flu. Complicating conditions must also be considered. The flu may be life-threatening for a person with emphysema, but only an annoyance for a healthy, 25-year-old. Despite its problems, the DRG system does take diagnosis and complicating conditions into account in setting payment rates for inpatient hospital care. Unfortunately, no classification scheme comparable to DRGs has yet been perfected for physicians' services generally or for outpatient care in particular.

One obvious solution would be to use the DRG system itself to determine physician payments. However, preliminary assessments (Mitchell, 1985) indicate that DRGs are not very good at predicting the costs of nonsurgical inpatient physician care and, thus, would need substantial refinement and modification before they could be used for reimbursing such inpatient physicians' services. The usefulness of DRGs in compensating for outpatient care is likely to be limited because they were developed to pay hospitals for inpatient services, not doctors or other providers for ambulatory care.

Policymakers can probably design solutions to some of these problems associated with paying for physicians' services prospectively on the basis of an illness episode. Suitable models for organizing physicians to receive Medicare payments could be developed and tested, methods that assure that the financial risks attendant to prospective payment schemes are spread among a large enough group of physicians so that the physicians' financial welfare would not be jeopardized. In addition, it may be feasible to design and implement a working definition of an episode of outpatient illness. It would be particularly important to define episodes clearly enough so that physicians would not be able to game the system by dividing a single incident into several, thus increasing his or her payment. Finally, policymakers may be able to define standards of care and mechanisms for monitoring physician practices that are sufficient to detect instances of undertreatment. The Health Care Financing Administration (HCFA) is hoping that the Peer Review Organizations (PROs) it has established to monitor its prospective payment system will be successful in preventing undertreatment of hospitalized patients. Perhaps PROs can form the basis of a comparable system for outpatient services.

Accomplishing these tasks, however, will require time and experimentation. In the meantime, the risks this option poses to quality of care provided Medicare patients would seem to outweigh its potential benefits in reducing Medicare expenditures.

Annual Payments

Another possibility, referred to as capitation, is a system under which a health care provider—either an individual physician or a health care organization—receives an annual sum to cover all the physicians' services required by a given Medicare beneficiary during the course of that year. The provider then assumes the financial risk entailed in taking responsibility for rendering these services. If the patient requires less care than expected, the provider makes money. If a catastrophic illness ensues, the provider may lose.

So that providers will be willing to assume such risks, the payment for each beneficiary must be adequate to pay for the physicians' services he or she is likely to require over the course of a year. Setting capitation rates is an actuarial problem. Beneficiaries would probably be classified on the basis of age, sex and possibly their disability status and prior medical history as well; an annual rate would then be calculated for each group of patients (adjusted, presumably, for the cost of living in the area of residence).

Most of the experience to date with capitated care has been with so-called fully capitated arrangements such as health maintenance organizations (HMOs), which assume responsibility for providing all the care patients may need, not just for physicians' services. Recently, Medicare began allowing beneficiaries to enroll in HMOs on a demonstration basis. The advantages and disadvantages of HMOs and other fully capitated arrangements for the Medicare population are discussed more completely in Chapter 7. Here we are concerned chiefly with the proposal that Medicare contract with organizations or individuals to provide physicians' services independently of other types of care.

The advantages of capitation are similar to those of lump-sum payments for an episode of illness. The physician or organization receiving the payment has no incentive to deliver unnecessary or marginally necessary services; and there are substantial incentives to find ways to deliver care more efficiently. An advantage compared to the episode-of-illness approach is that the unit of payment is clearly defined: a year of care. This makes the payment system much simpler from an administrative standpoint and much more difficult for physicians to manipulate to their own advantage. Payments would go out once a year (or monthly) from Medicare to each physician for each patient enrolled in his or her capitated group. Gone would be the requirement to define and to bill for each service or each episode of illness. Much paperwork would be eliminated and physicians could not break down the specified unit of service into smaller, billable units in the hope of increasing their income.

The major disadvantage of capitation is also similar to that of the previous option. Like all prospective payment schemes, capitation creates incentives to undertreat patients, with the sick particularly vulnerable. Individual physicians and organizations also have incentives to skim, or select, healthier patients in their enrollment process (Berenson, 1986). Medicare patients with chronic, costly illnesses could encounter difficulties with access to physicians' services. Though Medicare could legally require physicians to treat all comers and could monitor care for undertreatment (as it would have to do with an episode of illness approach), it would be costly and difficult to ride herd on the behavior of hundreds of thousands of physicians and tens of millions of patient-care episodes. The necessity to do so would detract from the administrative ease and cost-control potential of the capitation strategy.

Another drawback of capitating for physicians' services alone is that this approach may not be very effective compared with fully capitated arrangements in reducing health care expenditures. Most of the success experienced by HMOs in this regard has resulted from substituting outpatient physician care for more expensive hospital care. This option would not be available to individuals or organizations paid only for physicians' services.

A third problem with capitation approaches is that individual physicians may be placed at substantial financial risk if they were paid for all their patients on a capitated basis. A few very ill patients could create losses from which it would be difficult to recover. Because of these financial risks and because it constitutes such a radical change in the physicians' relationships with patients, the widespread or mandatory implementation of capitation payment is also likely to arouse substantial physician opposition.

Despite its drawbacks, the capitation strategy remains attractive because of the very positive past experience of fully capitated plans (albeit with non-Medicare patients for the most part) and the relative simplicity of administering such a scheme. More widespread experimentation with this option seems merited at the present time, with one important caveat: Medicare might want to consider contracting first with health care organizations (such as physician groups) rather than individual physicians in solo practice.

The reasons for this are several. Though there are no guarantees, even in groups, the tendency to undertreat the sick or skim the healthy patient may be reduced in situations where physicians interact frequently with colleagues who may observe their work. Also, groups may be able to spread the financial risks, so that physicians will feel less financially exposed and may be less inclined to cut treatment costs to the bone. Any widespread capitating of individual physicians for the provision of physicians' services should be undertaken only after mechanisms for monitoring patient selection and patient treatment are far more developed than they are at the current time.

Mandating Assignment

A final important issue in designing a method of paying physicians is whether the rate Medicare sets should be all the physician can receive for a given unit of care (i.e., whether assignment should be mandatory) or whether physicians should be permitted to seek additional compensation over and above the fee set by Medicare directly from patients. At least three options exist. First, physicians could be allowed to decide, as they currently do, whether or not to accept assignment separately for every unit of service they render.[4] Second, physicians could be required as a condition of participation in Medicare (i.e., in order for them or their patients to receive any payment) to accept assignment for all services (mandatory assignment). As a third, intermediate approach, physicians could be required to take assignment for all services or take it for none (the all-or-nothing approach). The difference between this and mandatory assignment is that Medicare would still be willing to reimburse patients who patronized physicians who refused assignment. Thus, all-or-nothing assignment forces physicians to accept Medicare payments as reimbursement in full or give up the option of ever billing Medicare directly, but it still subsidizes the provision of unassigned care by helping patients pay the bills.

Mandatory assignment has a number of advantages. It contributes to controlling societal health care costs by preventing physicians from eluding the payment limits established by Medicare. Requiring physicians to accept assignment also contributes to the program's fairness in certain respects by limiting the cost burden borne by beneficiaries, a burden that falls more heavily on the poor and on patients in geographic areas where, for whatever reasons, physicians are less likely to accept assignment. Mandatory assignment simplifies the Medicare program as well. Federal authorities no longer have to handle bills submitted by patients, which frequently do not contain necessary information. Physicians do not have to bill patients, and they deal exclusively with one payer (unless patients have supplementary insurance). Patients can more easily predict what they will actually have to pay for physicians' services, especially if mandatory assignment is combined with reforms that establish published fee schedules or prospectively determined lump-sum payments for episodes of illness.

Mandatory assignment, however, also has one main drawback: the threat of physician resistance. Unlike hospitals, many physicians could get by economically at the current time without seeing Medicare patients or, at least, without seeing as many as they currently see. Only seventeen percent of the average physician's earnings came from Medicare in 1981. (U.S. Congress, Senate, 1983; Levit et al., 1985). Forced to accept assignment, an unknown number of physicians might withdraw from participation in the Medicare program, thus creating a new barrier to access to services for beneficiaries. As we have seen, even the implementation of the all-or-none option could have a substantial effect on physician behavior. The more drastic step of mandatory assignment could seriously compromise access to services for particular specialties and in particular geographic areas. Such specialists include psychiatrists, orthopedic surgeons, gynecologists and ear, nose and throat (ENT) specialists, who currently derive relatively small amounts of their income from Medicare or deliver relatively small amounts of care on an assigned basis. Patients in rural localities with a relatively few oversubscribed physicians could face particular problems with access to care.

Policymakers should not be intimidated by the prospect of physician resistance to mandatory assignment. As the physician supply grows and as more private payers place restrictions on payment, physicians will have a harder time attracting patients, will become accustomed to limitations on their ability to set their own prices and will be more likely to accept Medicare restrictions on conditions of payment. Policymakers may want, therefore, to consider options that phase in tougher approaches toward assignment. The program could start with mandating assignment for hospital fees because physicians are currently more likely to accept assignment for hospital than outpatient services and, thus, effects on access to services would be minimized.

Hospital-Based Physicians

Certain specialists—notably radiologists, pathologists and anesthesiologists—are almost always based in hospitals and treat primarily hospitalized patients. They rarely have primary responsibility for the patient's care. At one time, most such physicians were employed directly by hospitals. Now, however, most such physicians are self-employed or are members of independent groups rather than salaried employees of hospitals.

Hospital-based physicians split off from hospitals because they could earn more by doing so. They could take advantage of the liberal reimbursement formulae of Medicare and other payers, and they no longer had to bargain with hospital authorities over salaries. The result, however, has been rapid escalation in the costs of services provided by hospital-based physicians.

To contain Medicare expenditures for this particular group of physicians it would seem logical to recognize explicitly that they provide services that are part and parcel of hospital care. This implies that payment for their services should be included in Medicare payments for hospital care (included as part of the DRG payment or factored into the hospital's target budget). This would immediately limit the rate of escalation in the cost of their services because they would no longer be paid on a fee-for-service basis and because hospitals would have an incentive to bargain carefully over their salary increases. Because both hospitals and other physicians have a pressing interest in the quality of care provided by hospital-based physicians, this change in economic incentives should not have an adverse effect on the quality of care for Medicare beneficiaries.

Conclusion

The question facing policymakers is not whether physician payment methods should be changed, but how. The way Medicare currently pays physicians has contributed to problems of cost, inequity and administrative complexity in the Medicare program. A number of options exist for reforming physician reimbursement. Among these, the development and implementation of a fee schedule based on relative values of services may be the most desirable in the next five years. Such a system could be used to reduce the escalation in physician expenditures, eliminate unjustified discrepancies in the amounts different physicians and services are reimbursed and promote policy goals such as redistribution of physicians to underserved areas. The implementation of a fee schedule would encounter less physician resistance in the short term, and politically it seems most feasible on a mandatory basis.

Over the longer term, experimentation should proceed with payment on a capitated basis. Although neither desirable nor feasible as a universal payment system at the current time, capitation is attractive for its cost-containment potential and its administrative simplicity. It may, however, have undesirable effects on quality of care and access to care, which require that it be implemented with caution.

A third option, reimbursement on the basis of episode of illness, faces severe technical problems in the short term. It has all the disadvantages of capitation and is likely to be administratively complex as well. Therefore, it seems the least desirable of the three general approaches.

The federal government should strongly consider the phasing in of mandatory assignment for physicians' services, starting with those provided in hospitals.

NOTES

1. By specialists, we mean chiefly physicians who have advanced training in a particular narrow field and see some or all of their patients on referral from other physicians. Examples include cardiologists, endocrinologists, dermatologists and thoracic surgeons. By primary

care physicians, we mean doctors who provide continuous, general care to patients. Examples include internists, general practitioners, family practitioners, and pediatricians.

2. Because it pays physicians less than other insurers, the Medicaid program has already encountered severe problems with physician resistance to treating Medicaid patients. In some areas, it is virtually impossible for Medicaid patients who are pregnant to find an obstetrician willing to treat them.

3. A recent study estimates that the average internist admits only 62 Medicare patients a year (Mitchell, 1985, p. 675).

4. That is, for every individual service, episode of illness or year of care.

REFERENCES

Andersen, Gerard F. and Jane E. Erickson. 1987. National Medical Care Spending. *Health Affairs* 6 (Fall):96–104.

Berenson, Robert A. 1986. Capitation and Conflict of Interest. *Health Affairs* 5(Spring):141–46.

Gornick, Marian, Jay N. Greenberg, Paul W. Eggers, et al. 1985. Twenty Years of Medicare and Medicaid: Covered Populations, Use of Benefits, and Program Expenditures. *Health Care Financing Review, 1985 Annual Supplement*, pp. 13–59.

Health Care Financing Administration, Office of the Actuary, 1986. Unpublished data.

Juba, David. 1985. *Decomposing Part B Payments for Physician Services.* Address to Health Care Financing Administration Symposium, *The Evidence on Medicare Physician Payment Alternatives*, Washington, January 16-17.

Levit, Katherine R., Helen Lazenby, Daniel R. Waldo, et al., 1985. National Health Expenditures, 1984. *Health Care Financing Review* 7 (1):1–35.

Medicine and Health. 1987. Physician Payments: Medicare's Next Battleground. Washington, D.C.: McGraw Hill. October 26, 1987.

Mitchell, Janet B. 1985. Physician DRGs. *New England Journal of Medicine* 313 (11):670–75.

Mitchell, Janet B., and Cromwell, Jerry. 1983. Impact of an All-or-Nothing Assignment Requirement Under Medicare. *Health Care Financing Review* 4 (4):59–78.

Pear, Robert. 1987. Plan for Medicare Forces U.S. to List Approved Doctors. *New York Times*, October 13:1.

Physician Payment Review Commission. 1987. Medicare Physician Payment: An Agenda for Reform. March 1, 1987.

Rice, Thomas. 1983. The Impact of Changing Medicare Reimbursement Rates on Physician-Induced Demand. *Medical Care* 21 (8):803–15.

Rice, Thomas, and Nelda McCall. 1982. Changes in Medicare Reimbursement in Colorado: Impact on Physicians' Economic Behavior. *Health Care Financing Review* 3 (4):67–85.

Tarlov, Alvin R. 1986. HMO Enrollment Growth and Physicians: The Third Compartment. *Health Affairs* 5 (1):23–35.

U.S. Congress. Office of Technology Assessment. 1986. *Payment for Physician Services: Strategies for Medicare.*

U.S. Congress. Senate. 1983. Committee on Finance and United States House of Representatives, Committees on Ways and Means and Energy and Commerce. *Background Data on Physician Reimbursement Under Medicare.*

U.S. Congress. Senate. 1984. Special Committee on Aging. *Medicare: Paying the Physician—History, Issues and Options.*

Wilensky, Gail R., and Louis F. Rossiter. 1983. The Relative Importance of Physician-Induced Demand in the Demand for Medical Care. *Milbank Memorial Fund Quarterly* 61 (2):252–77.

7

Medicare and Innovative Insurance Plans

MARK SCHLESINGER
PAMELA BROWN DRUMHELLER

Medicare was modeled on the private insurance available in 1965. At the time there was relatively little choice of insurance plans. Virtually all private health insurance paid for services in the same way, reimbursing treatment delivered by any licensed physician or accredited hospital on a fee-for-service basis.[1] Likewise, Medicare offered beneficiaries a fee-for-service plan with little choice of benefits (except the option to purchase Medicare Part B) and no choice of how health care providers would be paid.

The options available in private health insurance increased over the next two decades, particularly in recent years. Since 1980, about 20 million enrollees have switched from traditional insurance plans to prepaid plans (commonly called health maintenance organizations [HMOs]). In these plans providers are paid a predetermined amount for delivering all the health care an individual needs over the course of a year. Because providers are paid for each enrollee who joins the plan, these are sometimes called capitated plans. Many insurers also now offer preferred provider arrangements (PPAs) in which enrollees are strongly encouraged or required to use only those providers who have contracted with the insurer at discounted rates. Many working Americans can now choose among several different insurance arrangements, and the number and diversity of plans is likely to continue to grow in the future.

These changes in private insurance have sparked debate over the extent to which Medicare should offer its beneficiaries similar choices. In 1983, Congress authorized the Health Care Financing Administration (HCFA) to incorporate prepaid care into the Medicare program. More recently, legislators have proposed adding more options. Many policymakers believe that offering a range of plans gives Medicare beneficiaries the opportunity to select the one that best meets their needs and creates competition among insurers and providers that holds down health care costs. Others, though, are concerned that even if nontraditional insurance plans work well for younger Americans, they may be less suitable for the elderly. Experimental plans that are effective for private employers may also be less successful in Medicare.

In this chapter, we evaluate three alternative health insurance systems that have been, or are proposed to be, incorporated into the Medicare program. The first is prepaid care in health maintenance organizations. The second includes preferred provider arrangements and selective contracting with physicians. The third involves voucher plans that would replace the current Medicare program with one in which beneficiaries choose among a number of private insurance plans.

Health Maintenance Organizations

HMOs are paid in advance to provide a range of health care benefits, including at a minimum hospital and outpatient care. For the duration of the prepaid period, enrollees are covered only for those providers affiliated with the plan and those services authorized by the plan.

Unlike their counterparts in fee-for-service health care, providers in prepaid plans must work within a budget. This creates an incentive for them to conserve on the delivery of health services. Costs can be contained in a number of ways: substituting less costly for more expensive services, expanding the use of preventive care, better coordinating services to reduce inappropriate utilization and simply delivering fewer services. Because enrollees are covered only for services authorized by the plan, HMO physicians and administrators have more control over the services beneficiaries use. As a result, HMOs are thought to be better able as well as more motivated to efficiently manage health care services for their enrollees.

Apart from these common features, HMOs can take a variety of different organizational forms. Physicians may share a common office building, as do most prepaid group plans (PGPs), or practice out of individual offices, as in independent practice associations (IPAs). Some plans are federally qualified—that is, their coverages and organizational practices meet certain guidelines established by federal law in the mid-1970s—others are not. Some are operated by a small group of physicians or as physician-consumer cooperatives. Still others are a part of large national or multinational corporate systems.

Perhaps the most significant difference among prepaid plans is the extent to which individual physicians bear the financial consequences for the treatment of patients. Most early prepaid plans paid physicians primarily through a fixed annual salary (Meier and Tillotson, 1978). As a result, physicians faced little financial liability for patients who required costly treatment. More recently, an increasing number of plans base payment of physicians on the costs of treating their patients or all enrollees in the plan. For example, HMOs may deduct any costs of treating patients that exceed the average from their physicians' salaries. In the extreme, physicians may be individually capitated (i.e., paid a fixed amount per patient) and held financially liable for all their patients' health care expenses. Few plans to date have adopted complete physician capitation; most limit physicians' financial liability in one way or another.

A Growth Industry in Private Insurance

Over the past 10 years, HMOs of all types have become the fastest growing form of private insurance. In 1975, just under 6 million individuals enrolled in 178 HMOs. By mid-1985, there were 400 HMOs with 19 million enrollees (Interstudy, 1985). This rapid growth has been accompanied by some pronounced changes in the characteristics of the "average" HMO. IPAs are the fastest growing type of HMO; their share of total enrollment has tripled over the past decade. The proportion of enrollees in established HMOs (those in operation over 10 years) has fallen from 80 to 60 percent. Enrollment in federally-qualified plans has grown from under 50 to over 80 percent. Finally, large corporations are playing an increasing role in delivering prepaid care (Interstudy, 1985). In the mid-1970s Kaiser–Permanente operated the only major chain of HMOs; less than a dozen plans were owned by investors. By the mid-1980s there were 25 multistate HMO chains operating 150 plans; over a third of all HMOs were investor owned (Holmes et al., 1986). Perhaps the most significant change in the HMO industry has been the increased competition facing prepaid plans. As fee-for-service insurance programs have adopted various forms of preadmission screening and utilization review for hospitalization, they have become more competitive with prepaid plans (Goldsmith, 1984). As the number of HMOs has grown, so has the competition between them. The greater the amount of competition, the greater is the pressure on HMOs to hold down their costs (Schlesinger et al., 1986).

Delayed Acceptance Within Medicare

Although favored by the Nixon, Carter and Reagan administrations, HMO participation in the Medicare program was limited until fairly recently (Iglehart, 1985b). Some beneficiaries were enrolled in prepaid plans as early as the 1960s. But HMOs were reimbursed only for Part B services and were paid for whatever costs they incurred. Even after the 1972 Social Security Act amendments authorized prepayment for both Part A and Part B services, plans were subject to retrospective cost-based readjustments to their payments and a variety of restrictive regulations (Iversen and Polich, 1985). Because plans generally were uncomfortable with the need to maintain separate accounting systems for Medicare and for the rest of their enrollees, they did little to encourage Medicare beneficiaries to enroll (Iversen and Polich, 1985). As a result, by the end of the 1970s only several hundred thousand beneficiaries had joined HMOs, most because they had enrolled while working and stayed in the plan after retirement.[2]

Based on HMOs' track records in the private sector, though, congressional enthusiasm had begun to build. In the mid-1970s, HCFA was authorized to establish a series of demonstration projects in which Medicare beneficiaries joined prepaid plans on the same terms as younger enrollees. Enrollees in these demonstrations used less health care than the average elder in their community and were more satisfied with the quality of their care (Iversen and Polich, 1985).

Encouraged by the success of these demonstrations, in 1982 Congress amended the Social Security Act to expand Medicare enrollment in HMOs. The Tax Equity and Fiscal Responsibility Act (TEFRA) authorized that prepaid care be made available to all elders. Medicare beneficiaries were allowed to enroll both in federally qualified HMOs and in newly designated "competitive medical plans," which had to meet fewer federal requirements. Assuming that prepaid health care would be less costly, plans were paid for each enrollee at 95 percent of the average spending of a Medicare beneficiary of the same age and sex living in that community (the age/sex adjusted Medicare payment [AAPCC]). Plans with costs below these rates were required to offer additional benefits either through added coverage or reduced copayments. HCFA was instructed to supervise the marketing and enrollment practices of plans to ensure that any beneficiary who desired could join a participating HMO.

These amendments have been fairly successful in stimulating enrollment. As of June, 1986 (roughly one year after the final federal regulations were issued) 132 HMOs had agreed to participate, enrolling 630,000 beneficiaries on a prepaid basis (Iversen et al. 1985). Medicare enrollment in HMOs grew 40 percent between mid-1984 and mid-1985 and was predicted to increase by another 1.5 million by the end of 1987 (Ellwood, 1986).

Advantages/Disadvantages of Prepaid Care

Prepayment has become a part of Medicare. Some believe that this will greatly improve the program and that beneficiaries should be encouraged, or under certain conditions required, to join an HMO. Others fear that, in the long run, prepayment will present problems for both beneficiaries and the program itself. The evidence suggests that both positions have some merit. There are clearly immediate benefits for Medicare beneficiaries who enroll in prepaid plans. However, the long-term consequences for both the elderly and the Medicare program are less certain and more potentially problematic.

Expanded Coverage: Current Focus and Future Potential

To the extent that HMOs treat Medicare beneficiaries for less than the cost of care in a fee-for-service setting, Medicare regulations require that these savings be converted into added benefits for Medicare enrollees. The choice of which benefits to add to coverage is left to the HMO.

Most HMOs have chosen to either reduce copayments or cover ancillary medical expenses such as eyeglasses, dental care or prescription drugs (Iglehart, 1985b; Rossiter et al., 1985; Ellwood, 1986). These are important benefits. Copayments under the traditional Medicare program have become a major threat to beneficiaries' financial security (see Chapter 3). For many elders, particularly those with limited incomes, ancillary medical expenses are a major gap in Medicare's fee-for-service coverage (see Chapter 4).

A third option for enhanced HMO coverage is a prepaid plan that offers services to fill some of the current gaps in Medicare's coverage of long-term care (see Chapter 4). Interest in Congress has focused primarily on encouraging HMOs to substitute long-term services for those acute care services that are unnecessary or inappropriate.

> Bills introduced into the ninety-eighth Congress by home care proponents (such as Senators Packwood, Bradley and Helms and Representative Rangel) would

> provide a capitation payment identical to current Medicare costs but would permit the funds to be applied to currently uncovered long-term care services. This approach is in response to prevailing demand for cost-containment, but it permits expansion of long-term care services by shifting of funds now spent on presumably inappropriate acute care (Brecher and Knickman, 1985, p. 261).

The greatest potential for enhanced coverage in HMOs, however, may lie in the future. Although current savings in prepaid plans are too small to fund much additional long-term care (Brecher and Knickman, 1985), prepaid arrangements may offer the opportunity for expanding coverage. As discussed in Chapter 4, one of the major barriers to liberalizing Medicare's coverage of long-term care is the concern that this could lead to runaway program costs. If services are added in a prepaid setting, this is less likely to occur because the risks of cost overruns are shifted from program to provider. For this reason, Congress might be more willing to pay for expanded coverage of long-term care in prepaid settings than it has been in the past under fee-for-service reimbursement.

Cost Savings and the Paradox of Program Spending

Prepayment creates incentives for providers to limit health care use and thus hold down costs. Historically, costs of care for HMO enrollees have averaged 10 to 40 percent below costs for comparable populations treated under fee-for-service reimbursement (Luft, 1981; Manning et al., 1984). Most of these savings came from reduced rates of hospitalization.[3]

Because elders have much higher rates of hospitalization than younger patients, there was some initial concern that HMOs would be less able to contain costs for older enrollees. This concern proved to be unfounded. Although some plans have experienced high costs when first enrolling elders, both early Medicare enrollment in the 1970s (Weil, 1976) and Medicare's demonstration projects (Greenlick et al., 1983; Iglehart, 1985a) showed that HMOs were able to reduce hospitalization and the overall costs of treating the elderly. It is anticipated that savings will increase as HMOs begin to more actively compete with one another (Verway, 1985).

These cost savings will be even greater if HMOs enroll predominately healthy beneficiaries. HMOs may attract a healthier population for several reasons. First, because HMOs are at risk for expenses that exceed prepayment, plans have a financial incentive to enroll beneficiaries whose health care costs will be low. Plans can do this by selectively marketing to particular groups of elders who are likely to be healthier than average (Luft, 1982).[4]

Second, 90 percent of participating HMOs charge Medicare enrollees an additional premium to enroll in the plan: More than half exceed $250 a year and 15 percent charge more than $450 (Ellwood, 1986). The premiums pay for the costs of expanding Medicare coverage to the same breadth as that offered younger enrollees; typically plans prefer to avoid the complications caused by offering two sets of coverages to their members. High premiums, though, deter enrollment by elders who have little discretionary income. As a result, disproportionately wealthy—and as stastistics show, healthy—beneficiaries are the most likely to join prepaid plans.

Finally, past studies have found that individuals are more likely to join an HMO if they do not have an established relationship with a physician (Berki and

Ashcraft, 1980). Sicker individuals, particularly the chronically ill elderly, are more likely to have a regular source of medical care and thus are less likely to enroll in an HMO (Garfinkel et al., 1986).

Studies suggest that enrollees in HMOs do, in fact, tend to be unusually healthy. This has been true of both younger enrollees (Wilensky and Rossiter, 1986) and beneficiaries participating in several rounds of Medicare demonstration projects (Eggars and Prihoda, 1982; Garfinkel et al., 1986). The extent to which unusually healthy elders join HMOs, though, depends in part on the characteristics of the prepaid plan. For example, because IPAs use physicians practicing out of their conventional offices, elders do not need to switch doctors to join the plan. IPAs will therefore be less likely to attract only healthy elders without an established relationship with a physician.

Plans that place great financial risk on physicians, in contrast, will probably be associated with greater favorable selection because doctors can exert considerable influence over the enrollment or disenrollment decisions of their patients. In discussing HMO payment systems that make physicians financially responsible for the health care used by their patients, one physician noted, "Given these financial incentives, the best way to assure a satisfactory bottom line is to avoid seeing the sickest patients—the five percent who generate nearly half the costs. Thus, the physician's financial interest clearly requires him to encourage only his relatively healthy patients to sign up for the HMO (Berenson, 1986, p. 145)."

Thus, some of the ongoing changes in the HMO industry (e.g., greater financial incentives for physicians) will increase the likelihood of selective enrollment, whereas others (e.g., the increased role of IPAs) will discourage it.

Although enrollment of healthy beneficiaries results in broader coverage for these enrollees, it may create problems for the Medicare program. Paradoxically, even if HMOs reduce health care spending for every enrollee, the Medicare program will not necessarily realize any savings. Its costs may, in fact, increase.

This could occur if plans enroll beneficiaries whose costs would in any case have been less than 95 percent of the AAPCC in an area, the current Medicare payment rate for each beneficiary enrolled in an HMO. Medicare would then pay out more for these elders under prepayment than it would have under fee-for-service reimbursement. As a result of the various factors that encourage enrollment by healthier beneficiaries, this seems already to have happened. An ongoing study by the General Accounting Office (GAO) has preliminarily concluded that Medicare is overpaying HMOs by at least 5 percent owing to selective enrollment (*Hospital Week*, 1986). This is more than enough to offset savings produced by the 95 percent reimbursement rate, so that program costs may well be increased by beneficiaries' enrollment in HMOs.[5]

In an era of constrained governmental budgets, reforms that increase public spending are not likely to be viewed favorably. Selective enrollment could thus undermine political support for prepaid reforms under Medicare. It also raises questions about program fairness. Because Medicare requires that plans convert any surplus into additional benefits for enrollees, a program that overpays an HMO is indirectly subsidizing additional care for those who join the plan. Medicare beneficiaries joining HMOs tend to have above-average education and income and are healthier than the average elder (Eve and Reiss, 1981). If Medicare is going to spend more money, these funds could almost certainly be directed to beneficiaries with greater needs than those who join HMOs.

Nor are higher program costs the only potential problem created by selective enrollment. Even if most HMOs enroll unusually healthy elders, some may face the opposite situation. Particularly if organized as an IPA, HMOs may attract unhealthy patients. If this happens with the privately insured, the HMO can raise premium rates in subsequent years, offsetting their past losses. But this option is not available under Medicare, where prepayment rates are set by administrative formula. Plans that initially enroll high cost patients thus may face years of repeated losses from their Medicare beneficiaries. In relatively small plans, these losses may be financially catastrophic. To avoid this, they may be forced to drop out of the program.

Consequently, placing HMOs at risk for the cost of their Medicare enrollees also places beneficiaries at risk of losing their physician if the plan is forced to drop out of the program. At least one of Medicare's demonstration sites encountered this form of adverse selection, and the plan was forced to drop out of the demonstration (Eggars and Prihoda 1982). Telephone surveys conducted by Interstudy (a consulting firm specializing in the HMO industry) suggest that this is a growing concern for a number of plans now participating in the program.

Though these selection effects do not necessarily pose a direct threat to the welfare of beneficiaries, they create, in our assessment, enough significant problems for the program as a whole to merit some remedial actions. To limit these problems, the Medicare program would have to either discourage selective enrollment or better adjust HMO payments to reflect beneficiaries' expected use of health services or offer participating HMOs protection against significant financial losses. Reforms directed to each of these ends are discussed later in this chapter.

An Unclear Picture for Quality of Care

At this point, not enough is known about the quality of care in HMOs to reach any firm conclusions about their impact on enrollees' health (Luft, 1981). Recent studies of younger adults have found that outcomes of care for certain selected conditions are about the same in prepaid and fee-for-service settings, though low-income enrollees were found to be less healthy in an HMO than under fee-for-service care, whereas high-income enrollees fared better in prepaid settings (Yelin et al., 1985; Ware, et al., 1986).

Even less is known about the treatment of older enrollees. To date, the track record of HMOs participating in the Medicare program has been too limited to determine conclusively whether prepayment increases or decreases quality of care for the elderly. Some HMOs have developed case-management systems for Medicare enrollees (Iglehart, 1985b), but, as one recent assessment concluded, "most Medicare HMOs have fallen short of developing a health care delivery system that is well suited to the needs of the elderly" (Iversen and Polich, 1985). Medicare beneficiaries report that they are slightly more satisfied with care in prepaid plans (Ellwood, 1986), but there have been no good studies of health care outcomes to determine whether the care delivered is actually any different than in fee-for-service settings.

Not only is this evidence limited, but it is also based on the performance of the HMOs that participated in Medicare's initial rounds of demonstration projects. Many observers anticipate that differences between prepaid and fee-for-service care will become more pronounced as HMOs develop more experience with elder enrollees. Those who foresee benefits to enrollees believe that the organized structure and overall budget constraints of the HMO will encourage better coordinated care.

Others are concerned that the financial incentives and administrative arrangements in HMOs will lead to less adequate care for some elders.

More specifically, on the positive side, HMOs have potential for avoiding the biases toward inappropriate institutionalization that are now a part of the health care system. "The capitation plan creates incentives for the proper placement of institutional patients and would prevent, alleviate or retard the use of inpatient care when the services could be provided less expensively at home" (Winn and McCaffree, 1979, p. 187). Some policy analysts have also predicted that prepayment will encourage more preventive care, which is "particularly beneficial for older patients, whose decreased reserves and likelihood of compromising illnesses often result in less than optimal outcomes from late, heavily intensive intervention" (Bonanno and Wetle, 1984, p. 42).

On the negative side are two concerns. The first is that HMO-style health care will discourage effective patient management by physicians. Owing to their complex health needs, accurately diagnosing illness in the elderly is often a time-consuming, painstaking process (Rowe, 1985). Yet HMOs, particularly prepaid group practices, often limit the duration of physicians' appointments, leaving less opportunity for time-consuming diagnoses or communicating with patients than in fee-for-service practices (Luft, 1981).

A second concern is that the economic incentives produced by prepayment will discourage the treatment of chronic illnesses prevalent in the elderly (Schlesinger, 1986). An HMO has a financial incentive to expeditiously treat illness to avoid future costs to the plan. But the costs of most chronic illness are borne by the family of the elderly, not the HMO. Over 80 percent of all care for impaired elders come from family and friends (Manton and Liu, 1984; Doty, 1986). Prepaid plans thus have little financial incentive to treat many types of chronic illness.

Economic incentives, of course, are not the only factors influencing treatment and resource-allocation decisions. Professional standards obviously play a major role. However, here, too, patients with chronic illness are likely to be shortchanged in prepaid settings. There are few professional norms for treating the chronic conditions of the elderly, and such treatment ranks low on the hierarchy of professional prestige (Sapolsky, 1977; Pollack, 1979; Farrow et al., 1981) Under fee-for-service payment, there at least remains a financial incentive for continued treatment. Under prepayment, in contrast, physicians do not receive additional income for delivering additional services and, in fact, their incomes may decline as patients' costs go up.

The extent to which these various factors affect the health care of elders depends in part on the characteristics of the beneficiaries who enroll in HMOs. Elders with chronic illness are likely to be at a greater risk of adverse effects than are those with only acute diseases. Conversely, beneficiaries with complicated conditions requiring carefully coordinated services may well do better in prepaid plans.

The desirability of prepaid care for the elderly is also likely to be affected by the conditions facing the HMO. The evidence from Medicare's HMO demonstrations was based on the performance of a group of well-established plans operating under relatively uncompetitive conditions. Most plans currently participating in Medicare's prepayment program have far less experience; 40 percent have been in operation less than 5 years (Iversen et al., 1985). They are also facing more intense competition (Verway, 1985). Both of these factors are likely to squeeze HMOs' profits, putting them under greater pressure to decrease costs (Schlesinger et al., 1986). Inevitably, this puts elderly enrollees at greater risk of receiving inadequate care than they would be in a noncompetitive setting.

Given this possibility, the ability of the Medicare program to provide quality assurance for its beneficiaries in HMOs becomes an important issue. Currently, Medicare's HMO program contains two major safeguards against inadequate treatment. Unfortunately, neither is likely to prove fully effective.

First, there are regulations governing the types of services plans must offer. HMOs are required to offer a minimum package of benefits equal to those under fee-for-service coverage. Profiteering (excessive cost cutting leading to inadequate care) is discouraged by requiring that plans convert the surplus from treating beneficiaries into additional coverage.

Requiring that services be covered does not, however, ensure adequate utilization. HMOs use a variety of procedures to ration the services that are covered by the plan, including long waiting times for appointments and prior authorization for elective procedures (Luft, 1982). These controls, not coverage, become the principal determinants of health care use. For example, a recent report to the American Psychiatric Association included this assessment of mental health care in HMOs:

> The problem posed by HMOs was centered not so much on their lack of benefits coverage but on their limitations on service [such as refusal to accept mental health care referrals and administrative policies that discourage use of services]. . . . Access is often seen as being so restricted that care is nonexistent or is so limited that its effect is inconsequential (Mercer–Meidinger, 1986, p. 51).

As a second safeguard against inadequate treatment, Medicare requires that at least half the enrollment of participating HMOs be privately insured. This presumes that plans with inadequate quality will be unable to attract younger enrollees. As we have seen, however, many of the shortcomings of prepaid care may primarily affect the elderly. Younger enrollees may never experience these problems. As a result, the requirement that half the plans' enrollees be privately insured does not provide an adequate safeguard for appropriate treatment of Medicare beneficiaries. In fact, by discouraging plans from specializing, these provisions may encourage HMOs to downplay the special needs of older enrollees.

If quality of care for Medicare beneficiaries in HMOs is to be preserved, especially as competition among plans intensifies, better developed and more efficacious quality assurance methods must be established. A variety of alternatives are discussed next.

Options for Prepayment Reform

Prepayment under the Medicare program offers a number of important advantages for beneficiaries. Participating HMOs provide more comprehensive coverage of health care services and offer elders the opportunity to reduce their copayments in exchange for higher premiums. (Beneficiaries enrolled in prepaid plans thus avoid the need to purchase costly and often confusing Medigap policies to supplement their Medicare coverage.) The incentives produced by prepayment discourage unnecessary hospitalizations, improving both the quality and efficiency of elders' health care. In the end, prepaid plans may provide a vehicle for broadening Medicare's coverage of health care services to include long-term care.

As currently constituted, however, Medicare's prepayment system has two serious weaknesses. First, it is vulnerable to biased enrollment. Second, it does not adequately protect beneficiaries from the financial incentives of prepayment that could lead to undertreatment of certain illnesses. Reforms have been proposed to address each of these problems.

Reforms to Respond to Selective Enrollment

In principle, the most straightforward way for Medicare to avoid overpaying for beneficiaries would be to revise the AAPCC so that it accurately reflects what beneficiaries would have spent on health care had they stayed in the conventional Medicare program. In practice, predicting what beneficiaries' costs would have been is quite difficult. A number of promising options have been developed, many focusing on the amount of health care beneficiaries used in previous years (Thomas and Lichtenstein, 1986). Although these will undoubtedly improve the accuracy of the AAPCC, no formula developed in the near future is likely to accurately predict the future health care costs of Medicare's beneficiaries: too much depends on individual characteristics, needs and circumstances (McClure, 1984). As a result, the opportunity and incentive will still exist for HMOs to selectively enroll unusually healthy beneficiaries, or, conversely, to lose money if the plan inadvertently enrolls unusually sick elders.

Three approaches have been proposed for addressing the problem of selective enrollment. The first would standardize the marketing practices used by HMOs. The second would, under certain conditions, require that all beneficiaries join an HMO. The final option would partially shield HMOs from the high costs of an atypically unhealthy enrolled population.

Standardized Marketing Practices

Proposals that require more standardized marketing are a logical extension of current requirements that HCFA prevent discriminatory marketing and enrollment. Current regulations call for HCFA to oversee HMO marketing practices and to prohibit those that lead to selective enrollment. But this puts HCFA in the difficult role of assessing the effects of advertising practices. A more effective approach might be to establish guidelines that would promote less discriminatory marketing. Changes might include requiring (1) that benefits be marketed in a limited number of prototype combinations or (2) that the federal government include information about plans in Social Security mailings (Ginsburg, 1983).

By establishing a set of prototype benefit packages, HCFA could encourage enrollment of a more representative Medicare population. For example, participating plans could be required to offer a low-option coverage, one that would provide services and copayments that could be financed without requiring beneficiaries to pay an additional premium. This would limit the screening out of low-income elders.[6]

If the Social Security Administration distributed information about plans to all beneficiaries, the ability of HMOs to selectively market to low-cost enrollees would be limited.

> Having Medicare do the marketing of plans by informing beneficiaries of what plans were available in their area, and their prices, would reduce administrative costs substantially and avoid much preferred risk selection. With Medicare marketing the plans, opportunities for approaching only low-risk persons would be eliminated (Ginsburg, 1983, p. 115).

Such marketing reforms have one important side benefit. Under current arrangements, beneficiaries are likely to face a confusing choice of benefit packages offered by competing HMOs. Some elders will undoubtedly prove adept at selecting among prepaid plans, but others will have only limited understanding of the coverage they purchase (Greenfield, 1986). Standardized marketing of a more limited number of packages will make elders more informed purchasers. Those who understand their benefits are also more likely to pursue needed treatment, reducing the risk of underutilization.

The regulation of marketing has two potential drawbacks. First, by requiring that all plans select benefits from a set of prototype packages, regulations may stifle innovation. Yet, to date, most participating HMOs have shown very little interest in innovative coverages, adding only coverage for some ancillary medical expenses to basic Medicare benefits (Iversen and Polich, 1985). Rather than leaving innovation solely to the discretion of HMO administrators, it may prove more effective to foster experimentation through a series of demonstration projects such as those described later in this chapter. Successful experiments could subsequently be incorporated as additional options in the program.

Second, some critics fear that regulated marketing will hinder competition among plans, leading to less efficient delivery of health care (Havighurst, 1983). This seems unlikely. Socially beneficial competition can exist only if elders make knowledgeable choices among HMOs. By limiting choice to a small set of packages and by supplying beneficiaries with accurate information about plans, unadulterated by advertising hyperbole, standardized marketing reforms may lead to more useful and effective competition (Ginsburg, 1983). Even the most vociferous proponents of a competitive health care system acknowledge the need for government to act as an arbiter of the market (Enthoven, 1980).

There are some difficult questions about how best to regulate marketing practices. HCFA is now responsible for policing HMOs' marketing in a limited way, but this is an unfamiliar role. Oversight of marketing and advertising might better be assumed by agencies that have experience regulating advertising such as the Federal Trade Commission (FTC) or Federal Communications Commission (FCC).

Nevertheless, HCFA has experience dealing with health care markets, which have different characteristics than markets that the FTC and FCC traditionally monitor. In addition, it may be unwise to separate the roles of regulator and payer for services. Because HCFA reimburses participating HMOs and regulates enrollment, it could penalize plans that violate acceptable marketing practices by reducing payments or limiting future enrollment of Medicare beneficiaries. Another agency such as the FTC might have difficulty developing effective sanctions. It may be possible, however, that HCFA and the FTC could develop cooperative arrangements for policing marketing practices.

Mandatory Enrollment in HMOs

Several proposals would require that once a majority of beneficiaries in any community had voluntarily enrolled in prepaid plans, all elders in that community would be required to join an HMO (Sullivan and Samors, 1983; Friedman et al., 1984).[7]

Mandatory enrollment guarantees that program costs for the community will not increase as a result of selective enrollment because all beneficiaries must join some plan. This reform also has one important side benefit: It simplifies Medicare's regulatory requirements. A mixed fee-for-service and prepaid system requires that HCFA guard simultaneously against excessive utilization in the former and unjustified restrictions on access in the latter. Either of these is a major charge; to do both at once is especially difficult.

Mandatory enrollment, though, would also have some serious liabilities. To require that all elders join an HMO while continuing to allow younger Americans a choice between fee-for-service and prepaid care would be a retreat from the philosophy of mainstreaming the elderly. However great the potential or realized benefits of prepaid care, any plan that forces elders to join an HMO will inevitably raise the specter of second-class health care. This could undermine support for the program among both the elderly and younger taxpayers.

HMOs, moreover, will not necessarily be the best providers of health care for all beneficiaries. Enrollees who do best in prepaid settings are the ones who can negotiate their way through the administrative systems used to ration care (Luft, 1981). For others, and especially for elders who have chronic illnesses that may be undertreated in an HMO, the risks of prepaid care may outweigh the benefits. The HMO industry itself has been most sensitive to these limitations. Based on some early mixed experiences with Medicare enrollees, a number of HMO administrators have become convinced that some beneficiaries should be discouraged from joining prepaid plans. One HMO administrator concluded; "One of the few remedies available on HMOs is to educate Medicare members on provider procedures, restrictions and benefits. . . . They have to be told that HMOs are not for everybody" (Traska, 1986, p. 82).

Mandatory enrollment will not eliminate problems with selective enrollment for individual plans. HMOs will still have an incentive to select the least expensive enrollees. This has consequences for both beneficiaries and HMOs. Elders who are unusually sick and costly to care for may have trouble finding sources of care. Unable to fall back on a residual fee-for-service program, the sickest elders may become the least effectively treated, continually dumped from one HMO to another. Plans that enrolled a disproportionate number of such elders would find their costs exceeding their revenues and could eventually be forced out of business. Without precaution, an entirely prepaid system of care could thus be very unstable (McClure, 1984).

Finally, and perhaps most important, mandatory enrollment in HMOs runs counter to the principles of freedom of choice and pluralism that are characteristic of health care for other age groups. In the same way that HMOs have created competitive pressures that have encouraged fee-for-service insurers to hold down costs, the medical care delivered under fee-for-service auspices can provide standards for the adequacy of treatment in prepaid settings.

Reinsurance and Risk Sharing

Whether enrollment is voluntary or mandatory, HMOs have an incentive to selectively enroll healthy enrollees, and there is legitimate concern that they may, under some circumstances, enroll a sufficiently unhealthy population to suffer significant financial losses. One way to reduce the risks of this adverse selection and decrease incentives to compensate through favorable selection, would be to offer plans insurance against severe losses from serving the Medicare population. Most participating HMOs carry some form of private stop-loss insurance that covers them if spending on an individual enrollee exceeds $100 or $200 thousand dollars in a year. But this can still leave the plan exposed to significant risk if a number of elders have high utilization. HCFA could provide additional risk sharing by insuring against aggregate losses on a Medicare contract (Diamond and Berman, 1981).

This secondary insurance may reduce HMOs' incentives to hold down costs. But it would also reduce incentives that encourage plans to selectively market and to provide inadequate services to their chronically ill enrollees. This form of "partial capitation" may strike the best balance between incentives to maintain efficiency and quality of care (Greenberg et al. 1986).

Risk sharing issues also arise around proposals to capitate individual physicians for treatment of Medicare beneficiaries (Langwell and Hadley, 1986; U.S. Congressional Office of Technology Assessment, 1986). These proposals are intended to encourage the use of prepaid care in geographic areas where HMO's have been slow to develop. Unless carefully designed, however, they are likely to create financial pressures for those doctors who treat relatively sick elders—a physician's pool of patients is simply too small to allow adequate risk spreading. Physicians will thus have strong incentives to enroll patients selectively and will face financial pressures to limit treatment to the very ill. Some form of reinsurance or partial capitation would moderate these incentives and reduce the risks to elders.

Reforms to Protect the Quality of Prepaid Health Care

Two potential problems may affect the quality of prepaid care for the elderly. Prepayment creates incentives that may lead to inadequate treatment of chronic illness. Time pressures on physicians may also hinder diagnoses of complex disorders and discourage effective patient management. These problems are likely to become more pronounced as the market for prepaid care becomes more competitive and HMOs are under pressure to further cut costs.

There are three strategies for improving the quality of prepaid care for Medicare beneficiaries: (1) have HMOs cover a broader array of health and social services, (2) use a different strategy for regulating prepaid care, and (3) provide beneficiaries greater opportunities for appeal if they feel they have been denied adequate care.

Broadening Coverage in Prepaid Plans

Prepaid providers would deliver more appropriate care for chronic illness if the costs of untreated illness were borne to a greater extent by the HMO. Because many of these costs involve nonmedical services, one method of doing this is to include both medical and social services within the same prepaid plan.

Various forms of this strategy have been proposed in the academic literature—called social/health maintenance organizations (S/HMOs) or local area management organizations (LAMOs)—and there are ongoing demonstration projects to evaluate the feasibility of the S/HMO model (Ruchlin et al., 1982; Diamond et al., 1983; Iglehart, 1985b; Lentz et al., 1985). These plans combine funding from Medicare, Medicaid and various other programs financing social support services for the elderly under a single per capita rate.

It is too early to evaluate the results of these demonstrations. It is anticipated, however, that this approach will provide incentives for more appropriate care of the chronically ill because a S/HMO would bear more of the social costs of untreated illness. In addition, S/HMOs have the opportunity to substitute between medical and social services to reduce costs of care:

> Home health, personal care and social services are likely to increase due to improved systems controls in the S/HMO. . . . Of various long-term care reforms currently under consideration, the S/HMO offers the strongest possibility of centralized controls over patient management, and hence may offer the greatest potential for efficiency and cost savings (Diamond and Berman, 1981, p. 211).

Although this approach holds promise, S/HMO's ability to redirect resources to social services will be constrained by the amount of funding available for these services. Because the need for social services for the elderly has received less congressional attention than the need for medical services, programs such as Title XX of the Social Security Act and Title III of the Older Americans Act, which pay for social support services for the elderly, lack adequate funding. Few of the social support services needed to care for chronically ill elders are paid for through formal programs (Doty, 1986). Consequently, even if these programs paid for treatment in S/HMOs, there are not enough funds currently allocated to provide the services needed.

Despite this limitation, S/HMOs certainly have the potential for improving the health care of the elderly. However, it is important to be realistic about the extent to which organizational innovations alone, in the absence of more complete financing of social services, can provide the appropriate balance between social and medical services.

A Revised Approach to Regulation

In principle, Medicare's Peer Review Organizations (PROs) have responsibility for monitoring quality of care in prepaid plans as well as in the rest of the program. In practice, they have done relatively little. The HMO industry has resisted PRO review (Davis, 1985). Although the Reagan administration has asserted that HMOs should be reviewed by some organization other than a PRO (Traska, 1986), it recently acceded to Congressional pressures to initiate PRO review.

There is clearly a need for some external review of HMOs. Delegating quality assurance directly to the HMO creates great potential for conflict of interest. PROs, however, may not be the most appropriate agency to overview quality of care in prepaid settings. PROs have traditionally focused exclusively on hospital care and on relatively narrow medical criteria for that care. This perspective may not be suitable for assessing the behavior of HMOs, which provide a broad array of inpatient and outpatient services.

Whatever the mechanism, some form of more active oversight of HMO performance is almost certainly merited. The current approach to regulating Medicare

HMOs has placed HCFA in a relatively passive role, establishing a set of simple criteria that the plans must meet: coverage must be at least equal to that offered under Medicare's fee-for-service program; half of all the plan's enrollees must be privately insured; any of the money from Medicare reimbursement not spent on basic services must be reinvested in added coverage or reduced copayments. The criteria are easily specified and readily monitored. Unfortunately, they cannot in themselves assure adequate treatment for the elderly.

As noted earlier, requiring that services are covered does not guarantee that they will be actually made available because HMOs ration care in a variety of ways. Enrollment by younger, privately insured individuals does not ensure that the special health care needs of the elderly are being met. Similarly, requiring that plans spend their surplus on added benefits does not protect the elderly from profiteering plans. Profits can readily be disguised as costs: Administrators can be paid excessively high salaries, and large fees can be paid to subsidiaries ostensibly supplying services to the HMO (Goldberg, 1975; Etzioni and Doty, 1976). To provide true safeguards against profiteering at the expense of Medicare beneficiaries, HCFA or some other agency must have the power and resources to periodically audit prepaid providers.

More generally, it may be more effective to monitor the actual performance of participating plans than to construct regulations to guard against potential problems. More active monitoring would require that PROs, or a similar agency, play an active role in supervising HMOs (Traska, 1986). It would also probably require a set of sanctions that could be imposed on plans that were inadequately caring for beneficiaries. Currently, the only real sanction is to withdraw certification from participating HMOs. HCFA has been hesitant to employ this penalty. Throwing plans out of the program entirely could damage the reputation of the program. It could also disrupt continuity of care for beneficiaries enrolled in the plan (Sorian, 1986). Providing HCFA with more alternatives for imposing financial penalties on HMOs would create a financial incentive for plans to improve their performance without disrupting the program or the health care of beneficiaries.

Putting a greater emphasis on monitoring HMOs' performance would have an important advantage. A number of existing criteria such as the requirement that 50 percent of an HMO's enrollees be privately insured were created as indirect protections for quality of care under the assumption that more direct measures were not feasible or appropriate. As better measures of quality are developed in the future, these indirect safeguards can be eliminated or relaxed, giving plans greater flexibility and potentially improving the quality of delivered services. For example, allowing HMOs to enroll primarily elderly patients would permit them to specialize in geriatric care and develop service systems designed to meet the special needs of the elderly. This reform also might encourage agencies with expertise in health care for the elderly such as geriatric facilities and home health care agencies to establish HMOs (Bonnano and Wetle, 1984).[8]

To ensure that Medicare beneficiaries receive good quality care in prepaid settings, more active monitoring of HMOs should be phased in over time.[9] This could begin with audits of how Medicare revenues are spent within prepaid plans to determine if revenues are related to the actual costs of treating enrollees. Priority should be given to developing standards of appropriate access for the care of chronic illness among the elderly. These could be used in future assessments of the performance of plans participating in Medicare's prepayment program.

Increased Opportunities for Grievance Procedures

A third option for improving care of the elderly in HMOs is to provide beneficiaries with a greater opportunity to appeal if they feel that they have been denied adequate care. Currently, Medicare's HMO arrangements are based on a traditional competitive model—if beneficiaries are dissatisfied with a particular HMO, they are expected to switch to another that better meets their needs (Enthoven, 1978). But many elders place a high priority on maintaining an established relationship with a particular doctor (Garfinkel et al., 1986; LaTour et al., 1986). This makes them reticent to switch plans.

Because leaving a plan is difficult for elders, one alternative is to provide them with greater opportunity to voice their concerns (Hirschman, 1970). After investigating some emerging problems with participating HMOs in Florida, both the GAO and the inspector general of the Department of Health and Human Services (DHHS) concluded that beneficiaries needed clearer guidelines for grievances and appeals (Firshein, 1986; *Hospital Week*, 1986). These could be incorporated into the existing Medicare appeals process or made a function of a separate ombudsman agency (Kerschner, 1986).

Creating more options for registering appeals and complaints would provide HCFA with a source of information for evaluating the performance of the evolving HMO industry. This approach also has advantages over regulation. It is less likely to inhibit innovative arrangements for providing care and, because appeals would be initiated by beneficiaries, it offers opportunities to respond to those issues that are of greatest concern to the elderly.[10]

Perhaps the most serious drawback with an enhanced appeals process is that it relies on elders' willingness to make a complaint. A substantial number of the elderly do not seek care from a doctor when they feel ill, assuming symptoms to be merely a natural part of growing old (Branch and Nemeth, 1985; Rowe, 1985). If elders are told by an HMO that they do not need care, they may be all too willing to accept this assessment rather than question physician decisions.

If a grievance system is to be an effective safeguard against undertreatment, it must be coupled with a program of patient advocacy and beneficiary education. The elderly must become better informed purchasers of health care, able to assess to a greater extent when they should seek medical advice (Somers, 1984). If successfully implemented, such a combined program could provide a useful complement to regulatory limits on undertreatment because beneficiaries are likely to be sensitive to aspects of quality that may be difficult to formalize as regulatory criteria.

Preferred Provider Arrangements

Medicare as Selective Purchaser of Health Services

In the past five years, a second innovation has become increasingly common in private insurance. Termed preferred provider arrangements (PPAs) or organizations (PPOs), these incorporate two functions not found in conventional fee-for-service insurance plans (Lissovoy et al., 1986). First, the insurer selectively contracts with a limited number of hospitals and physician groups. Providers agree to offer care at discount prices; in exchange, the insurance plan creates financial incentives for enrollees to use these providers.[11] Second, extensive utilization review is built into the plan—over 90 percent of all PPAs require prior authorization by the insurer for selected hospital treatments; almost as many plans include concurrent reviews of hospital stays (Rice et al., 1985).

Although PPAs are a fairly recent innovation, they are growing rapidly (Gabel and Ermann, 1985). Virtually nonexistent in 1980, there were over two hundred plans operating by 1985 (American Medical Care Review Association, 1985). The number of privately insured individuals eligible to join a PPA grew fourfold between 1984 and 1985 (Rice et al., 1985). A number of states, including Arizona, California and Illinois, have incorporated selective contracting into their Medicaid programs.

Similar arrangements have been proposed for Medicare beneficiaries (Ginsburg, 1983).[12] Medicare could selectively contract with a limited number of providers, perhaps using a competitive bidding process to identify low-cost hospitals or physician groups. Beneficiaries would be required to use these providers or else pay an additional copayment (equal to the difference between the PPA's discount prices and the charges of the providers that the beneficiary used). More extensive utilization review would be incorporated into the plan. Savings could be split between the program and participating beneficiaries who would pay a reduced premium.

The PPAs are thought to have two major advantages over Medicare's traditional insurance system. First, by selectively contracting and negotiating prices, preferred provider systems may lower program costs and, thus, beneficiaries' premiums. Both private PPAs and states' Medicaid programs have been able to negotiate prices 10 to 15 percent lower than they had paid previously (Christianson et al., 1983; Friedman, 1984; Rice et al., 1985). Second, more extensive utilization review may improve quality by reducing inappropriate utilization (Greenberg, 1983).

The benefits of a PPA, however, are likely to be smaller for Medicare than for private insurers. Because Medicare pays for a significant portion of health care in this country, the program has substantial bargaining power to negotiate lower rates even without selective contracting. Studies have found, for example, that Medicare pays 19 to 20 percent less than do commercial insurers for a stay in the hospital (Sloan and Becker, 1984; Davis and Rowland, 1986). This is larger than the average discount negotiated through a PPA. There may not, therefore, be much opportunity for negotiating further reductions in hospital payments.

Greater opportunities may exist for savings in physician reimbursement (see Chapter 6). Medicare, however, may be able to capture much of this saving by requiring mandatory assignment (creating, in effect a quasi PPA) without the administrative costs of a more formal preferred provider system.

Nor would PPAs' utilization review represent a great advance for Medicare. Medicare already has a form of utilization review incorporated into its PROs. Although these focus only on hospital care, this is also true of much of the utilization review in PPAs. Surveys have found that although over 90 percent of the private preferred provider systems have some form of utilization review for hospitalization, only a quarter review outpatient utilization (Rice et al., 1985). To the extent that private systems develop effective means of utilization review, it may be more sensible and less administratively cumbersome to simply incorporate these into PROs rather than establish de novo a preferred provider system for elder enrollees.

Not only are PPAs likely to offer fewer advantages for Medicare than for other payers, but the liabilities may be greater as well. Selective contracting creates particular problems for the elderly. First, asking enrollees to pay an additional copayment if they receive care from a nonpreferred provider adds yet another form of cost sharing to an array of copayments and deductibles that is already excessive (see Chapter 3).

Second, to ensure that enrollees actually use contracted providers, a number of private PPAs have found it necessary to go beyond simply offering financial incentives for using particular providers—enrollees are locked-in to preferred providers and treatment from other sources is not reimbursed (Traska, 1986). The undesirable effects of such a lock-in would probably be greater for Medicare beneficiaries than for younger individuals. Many elders have limited mobility, making it difficult for them to reach providers located far from their home (Iversen and Polich, 1985). If Medicare were to contract with only a few hospitals and physician groups in a community, some beneficiaries would find it difficult to obtain needed care.

Finally, contracting by a public agency such as HCFA is often more complicated and less flexible than contracting by private organizations. Providers may be able to exert considerable political pressure to get or maintain a Medicare contract. As we have learned all too well from the Department of Defense's experience, a public agency purchasing services may become more concerned with preserving the financial stability of contractors than with obtaining services of good quality or low cost (Schlesinger et al., 1986). Thus, although selective contracting in a public program may produce cost savings in the short term, it may actually lead to poorer performance in the long run.

Beneficiary Choice and a Voucher System

In recent years, policymakers have sought to introduce more competition into the health care system. Their preferred approach has been to offer the insured a variety of plans to choose from.

> The common denominator of the major competition bills, including those that provide for vouchers for individuals enrolled in Medicare and Medicaid, is that insurer-based competition—that is, among third-party insurers, alternative delivery systems, limited-provider groups and health maintenance organizations (HMOs)—is the most viable, if not the only, form of competition in health care (Greenberg, 1983, pp. 46–47).

To expand choice and enhance competition within the Medicare program, it has been proposed that beneficiaries be given a voucher of fixed value to purchase a year's worth of insurance coverage from a private insurer. Voucher systems appeared in a half-dozen bills introduced to Congress in the early 1980s. Throughout this period, virtually every major Medicare reform proposal incorporated vouchers in one form or another.[13]

A voucher system, it is argued, has several advantages over the current Medicare system. First, it would allow beneficiaries to cash in the portion of their voucher they did not use to purchase insurance (Firshein, 1986). This, it is predicted, will induce beneficiaries to be more conscious of costs when selecting an insurer, creating competitive pressures that will hold down program expenditures (Babbitt and Rose, 1986). Second, a voucher system allows beneficiaries greater choice in selecting the types of services they wish covered.

> Implicit in the competition advocate's message is the idea that there is no single right way to organize health care delivery or to treat particular diseases and that, with accountability to consumers ensured in the marketplace, decisions on such sensitive and significant matters can be safely entrusted to private actors (Havighurst, 1983, p. 29).

Allowing beneficiaries choice has considerable intuitive appeal. Given the historical difficulties in generating a political consensus to improve Medicare's coverage of services, permitting beneficiaries the option to select their own insurance coverage seems promising. It is less apparent, however, that increasing the number of options beyond those that already exist would necessarily benefit Medicare's enrollees.

Beneficiaries currently have the option to choose between fee-for-service coverage and a number of prepaid plans. The pertinent question is thus whether they gain much if these options are expanded. A voucher system would offer three additional choices: the ability to cash in a portion of the voucher; the option to choose a private, fee-for-service insurance plan; or the option to select a private PPO.

It seems quite unlikely that many elders would cash in a portion of their voucher. Very few elders want less insurance coverage than Medicare provides; currently, about 80 percent of the elderly not covered by Medicaid purchase private insurance policies that supplement Medicare, and those who do not are not able to afford the policies (Hagen, 1986). Because few elders would trade insurance benefits for cash, creating a cash-back option would not make elders as a group more cost conscious and, thus, would not lead to any significant reductions in program costs.

Nor does it seem likely that many beneficiaries would choose private fee-for-service insurance over the traditional Medicare program. Private insurance is simply a bad buy. The costs of administration and marketing for private plans are much higher than the administrative costs of the Medicare program: The former run between 30 and 40 percent of the value of premiums for policies marketed to individual elders; the latter about 3 percent (Davis and Rowland, 1986).[14] The prices paid by private insurers for hospital and physician services are also significantly higher than those paid by Medicare (Sloan and Becker, 1984; Cromwell and Burstein, 1985). Because private insurers have higher costs for administration and per unit of service, they generally cannot offer, for a voucher of given value, as comprehensive coverage as can the Medicare program.

The third alternative involves giving beneficiaries the option to use private PPAs. Private PPAs may offer some advantages over a PPA sponsored by Medicare. Private contracting may avoid some of the political constraints that hinder effective contracting by a public agency. Selective contracting would allow private insurers to negotiate lower prices, offsetting some of their cost disadvantage compared to the Medicare program. Still, the added administrative costs of private insurance and the disadvantages of plans limited to a small number of providers are likely to make PPAs attractive to only a few of the elderly.

It therefore appears that only a small number of beneficiaries would gain from the additional options provided by a voucher system. These restricted benefits must be weighed against costs that would be borne by the program as a whole and by all beneficiaries. A Medicare system based on vouchers would have three major liabilities. First, such a system would face the same problems of selective enrollment as does Medicare's current prepaid system. If only healthier beneficiaries purchased private insurance with their vouchers, the Medicare program could become more expensive (Ginsburg, 1983). Since private insurers have strong financial incentives to selectively market policies, this is quite likely to occur.

Second, for many beneficiaries, adding options will only create complexity and confusion. Though some beneficiaries would undoubtedly be willing and able to choose among a variety of plans, many elders have difficulty understanding the provisions of the traditional Medicare program (McCall et al., 1986). Introducing the option of prepaid care has compounded this confusion (Greenfield, 1986; Kerschner, 1986). It would be increased yet again if elders also had to choose among a number of private fee-for-service insurers and PPAs. Further, based on the track record of insurers marketing Medigap policies, it is likely that the advertising of these private policies will do more to cloud than clarify the choices beneficiaries must make (DeNovo and Shearer, 1978; Hagen, 1986).

Finally, introducing vouchers would fragment the Medicare program, making it increasingly difficult to administer. Quality assurance programs would need to be adapted to each of the different sets of incentives created under different models of selective contracting, utilization review, and prepayment. Appeals processes would have to be established to deal with many hundreds of different private insurance plans.

Perhaps equally important, fragmentation could affect the political support for the program. It has been difficult to create political consensus to improve the Medicare program. Improvements could become impossible if there were not one Medicare program, but hundreds of different programs, each associated with a different private insurer. This is particularly true if younger, wealthier, more politically active beneficiaries choose to join private plans, leaving those with the fewest resources in the traditional Medicare program (Firshein, 1986).

Incorporating Innovative Insurance Systems into the Medicare Program

It is important that public programs like Medicare remain flexible enough to respond to ongoing changes in the health care system. To this end, the private insurance industry provides a useful standard of comparison. As we have seen, however, not all that works well for younger enrollees of private insurance plans can be readily transferred to older beneficiaries of a public insurance program. Some innovations must be tailored to the special needs of the elderly. Others probably cannot be adapted sufficiently to make them worthwhile additions to the Medicare program.

Whatever one concludes about specific insurance arrangements, however, there are some general issues that cut across all potential innovations. We have touched on these in the course of our discussion, but it seems useful to emphasize them.

How Much Choice Is Appropriate?

As private insurers adopt alternative arrangements, Medicare will be pressured to do the same. Those who are concerned with frugality will argue that Medicare should be just as aggressive as the private sector in trying to cut costs. As we have seen, although these plans may be less costly for the beneficiaries who enroll, they may increase costs to the Medicare program.

Others will argue for innovation in the name of equity, believing that Medicare beneficiaries should have as many choices open to them as are available to younger Americans. However, in this case, more is not necessarily better. Introducing too many options can make the program so confusing that many beneficiaries are unable to choose wisely. The confusion in itself can undermine elders' confidence in the program and their peace of mind. No doubt some beneficiaries would prosper if given the choice of a broad array of plans. Others can be made more aware of their options, made better-informed consumers. But there are limits to this improvement and there is real value for the majority of elders in having a program that is simple and easy to comprehend.

Introducing new options also tends to fragment the program. This can lead to selective enrollment of elders in particular types of plans, potentially increasing program costs. A fragmented program would thus be less effective as an insurance program, less able to spread risks between sick and healthy elders. Medicare may also lose political strength, particularly if the elders with the greatest political voice gravitate to one part of the program, leaving others to an inadequately supported and insufficiently funded residual program.

Finally, adding alternative systems increases the administrative burdens on the Medicare program. As we have seen, no method of paying providers or organizing insurance is a panacea; each creates new problems even as it remedies old ones. Consequently, public oversight and regulation will always be an important part of the Medicare program. Effectively assuring that quality and access are maintained can be a daunting proposition under any single insurance or payment system. With each newly introduced system, the problems of oversight are compounded.

At what point the Medicare program becomes too complex for beneficiaries to effectively use, or for administrators to efficiently oversee, is something that should be thought about carefully. Medicare is already so complicated that adding insurance plans, such as PPOs, will make the program less rather than more effective.

How Should Innovations Be Incorporated Into Medicare?

If Congress concludes that there is still room in Medicare for further innovation, the question of how new insurance arrangements should be implemented remains. As we have seen, the health care needs of the elderly are significantly different from those of younger individuals; the strengths and weaknesses of a public program differ from those of private enterprise. As a result, one cannot simply borrow what seems to be working well for private insurers. It therefore seems wise to continue to use the approach developed for introducing prepaid care to Medicare: begin with a series of demonstration projects through which the basic principles of the innovation can be fine-tuned to the needs of the program and its beneficiaries.

If this experimentation is to prove effective, however, it is important that the types of plans involved in the demonstrations be reasonably representative of those that are likely to later be incorporated into the program as a whole. By this criteria, Medicare's assessment of HMOs has fallen short. As described earlier, the plans that have chosen to participate in Medicare's HMO program are very different from those that were involved in the initial demonstration projects. Participating HMOs are less well established, more likely to be independent practice associations and more likely to be operated for profit (over half of all enrollees in plans with at-risk contracts are in for-profit HMOs) (Iversen et al., 1985).

We do not yet know if the performance of these HMOs will live up to the experience of those involved in the demonstration projects. It seems most unwise, however, to have assumed that one HMO would be much like another or that plans with a very limited track record and under different organizational auspices would necessarily perform as well as their predecessors. More generally, if demonstration projects are to be effective tests of innovative insurance arrangements, they should evaluate the types of plans that will actually participate in the program.[15] As innovative arrangements evolve over time, new experiments should be conducted to reevaluate their performance.

Finally, however effective the demonstration process, it is essential that careful oversight be maintained as innovations are added to the program. This does not mean that we should attempt to preempt problems through a web of regulation. The regulatory burden must be kept tolerable to encourage participation and innovation. It does require, though, that effective mechanisms be put in place to identify when beneficiaries are not being well served. Another of the early lessons from Medicare's prepaid system was that HMOs were brought into the program before such safeguards were established, and some beneficiaries suffered as a result (Ellwood, 1986).

These safeguards could take the form of provider audits, more extensive appeals processes or local Medicare ombudsmen's offices that could identify beneficiaries' concerns. Whatever their form, it is essential that those administering the Medicare program be as sensitive to the liabilities of innovative payment and insurance arrangements as they have become to the shortcomings of Medicare's traditional fee-for-service program. Given this awareness, we anticipate that a number of innovation insurance arrangements can be adapted to the needs of beneficiaries and the goals of the program as a whole.

NOTES

1. Under fee-for-service reimbursement, providers are paid a separate fee for each visit, service or procedure.

2. A small number of beneficiaries participated in a half dozen demonstration projects in which Medicare paid HMOs for services on a prepaid basis.

3. In the past several years, hospitalization in the health care system as a whole has been steadily declining, but it has remained roughly constant in prepaid groups (Boston Consulting Group, 1984). As a result, HMOs' cost advantage has shrunk, though it is difficult to determine exactly by how much.

4. Although the Health Care Financing Administration is required to police marketing practices, proving that advertising is intended to attract low-cost enrollees would be almost impossible.

5. This problem is not unique to Medicare. Recent surveys indicate that 60 percent of private employers believe that health maintenance organizations (HMOs) have either increased or left unchanged their health care costs (Taylor and Kagay, 1986).

6. Fifteen percent of participating plans now offer coverage with no added premiums, suggesting that this requirement would be financially feasible.

7. This includes a plan sponsored by David Stockman when he was in Congress.

8. Loosening or eliminating the 50 percent enrollment restriction has been favored by both the Reagan administration and influential members of Congress (Traska, 1986; Iglehart, 1985a).

9. Prospects for loosening the 50-percent restriction were recently dealt a serious political blow. One of the two health maintenance organizations (HMOs) currently operating under waivers allowing for more than 50-percent Medicare enrollment became the target of several federal investigations. These revealed a number of practices that violated Medicare regulations. As a result, Congress has become far more wary of loosening enrollment restrictions and is not likely to do so in the immediate future (Firshein, 1986).

10. It would be important to develop ways to convert complaints into remedial action. Past efforts to incorporate ombudsmen into programs paying for nursing home care have used the ombudsman's office as a means of gathering information that is then passed on to regulators.

11. Typically, enrollees pay only limited copayments if treated by a provider with a contract, but they must pay more if they seek care from other providers.

12. To date, most of the proposals for introducing preferred provider arrangements to Medicare have been part of more ambitious group capitation plans. Under these plans, administration of the Medicare program would be transferred to a private agency for a defined set of beneficiaries. For example, the Reagan administration has considered transferring administration of the Medicare program in Maryland to the Blue Cross/Blue Shield plan in that state. Chrysler has proposed assuming administration of the plan for its retired workers (Rich, 1986). These private administrators would then make available to beneficiaries a range of coverages, including HMOs, fee-for-service coverage and preferred provider organizations.

13. These are reviewed briefly in Davis and Rowland (1986) and Schlesinger (1986).

14. Even if policies were marketed through groups such as the American Association of Retired Persons (AARP), they would have administrative and marketing costs several times as large as those of the Medicare program (Blair and Vogel, 1975).

15. Alternatively, it may be desirable to limit HMO participation in the Medicare program to those insurance plans with characteristics like those that participated in the original demonstration projects. For example, participation might be limited to only HMOs with some minimal track record. Under the regulations for HMO participation initially incorporated into the Medicare program in 1972, for example, plans were required to have been in operation for at least three years before enrolling Medicare beneficiaries (Iversen and Polich, 1985).

REFERENCES

American Medical Care and Review Association. 1985. *Directory of Preferred Provider Organizations and Industry Report on PPO Development*. Bethesda, MD.

Babbitt, B., and J. Rose. 1986. Building a Better Mousetrap: Health Care Reform and the Arizona Program. *Yale Journal on Regulation* 3 (2):243–82.

Berenson, R. A. 1986. Capitation and Conflict of Interest. *Health Affairs* 5(1):141–46.

Berki, S. E., and M. L. F. Ashcraft. 1980. HMO Enrollment: Who Joins What and Why: A Review of the Literature. *Milbank Memorial Fund Quarterly* 58 (4):588.

Blair, R., and R. Vogel. 1975. *The Cost of Health Insurance Administration.* Lexington, MA: Lexington Books.

Bonanno, J., and T. Wetle. 1984. HMO Enrollment of Medicare Recipients: An Analysis of Incentives and Barriers. *Journal of Health Politics, Policy and Law* 9(1):41–62.

Boston Consulting Group, 1984. *HMO Report.* Boston: Schlesinger.

Branch, L. G., and K. T. Nemeth. 1985. When Elders Fail to Visit Physicians. *Medical Care* 23 (11):1265–75.

Brecher, C., and J. Knickman. 1985. A Reconsideration of Long-Term-Care Policy. *Journal of Health Politics, Policy and Law* 10 (2):245–73.

Christianson, J., D. Hillman and K. Smith. 1983. The Arizona Experiment: Competitive Bidding for Indigent Medical Care. *Health Affairs* 2 (3):88–103.

Cromwell, J., and P. Burstein. 1985. Physician Losses from Medicare and Medicaid Discounts: How Real Are They? *Health Care Financing Review* 6 (4):51–68.

Davis, C. K., 1985. Medicare Risk Contracts—A Challenge Worth Meeting. In *HMOs Confronting New Challenges, June 1985.* Conference Proceedings, Annual Meeting of Group Health Association of America, pp. 5–170.

Davis, K. and D. Rowland, 1986. *Medicare Policy: New Directions for Health and Long-Term Care.* Baltimore: Johns Hopkins University Press.

DeNovo, A., and G. Shearer. 1978. *Private Health Insurance to Supplement Medicare,* Volume 1. Policy Planning Issues Paper. Federal Trade Commission.

Diamond, L. M., and D. E. Berman. 1981. The Social/Health Maintenance Organization: A Single-Entry, Prepaid Long-Term-Care-Delivery System. In *Reforming the Long-Term-Care System,* ed. J. J. Callahan, Jr., and S. S. Wallack, pp. 185–218. Lexington, MA: Lexington Books.

Diamond, L., L. Gruenberg and R. Morris. 1983. Elder Care for the 1980s: Health and Social Service in One Prepaid Health Maintenance System. *Gerontologist* 28:143–54.

Doty, P. 1986. Family Care of the Elderly: The Role of Public Policy. *Milbank Quarterly* 64 (1):34–75.

Eggars, P. W., and R. Prihoda. 1982. Pre-enrollment Reimbusement Patterns of Medicare Beneficiaries Enrolled in 'At-Risk' HMOs. *Health Care Financing Review* 4 (1):55–73.

Ellwood, D. A. 1986. Medicare Risk Contracting: Promise and Problems. *Health Affairs* 5 (1):183–89.

Enthoven, A. C. 1978. Consumer-Choice Health Plan. *New England Journal of Medicine* 298 (12):717–22.

———. 1980. *Health Plan.* Reading, MA: Addison Wesley.

Eve, S., and E. Reiss. 1981. Use of Health Maintenance Organizations by Older Americans. Paper presented at the 34th Annual Scientific Meeting of the Gerontological Society of America, Toronto, Canada, November 8–12.

Etzioni, A., and P. Doty. 1976. Profit in Not-for-Profit Corporations: The Example of Health Care. *Political Science Quarterly* 91 (3):431–53.

Farrow, F., T. Joe, J. Meltzer et al. 1981. The Framework and Directions for Change. In *Policy Options in Long-Term Care,* ed. J. Meltzer, F. Farrow, and H. Richman, pp. 1–37. Chicago: University of Chicago Press.

Firshein, J. 1986. No Ground Swell of Support for Voucher Plan. *Hospitals* 60:24–26.

Friedman, B., S. A. LaTour and E. F. X. Hughes. 1984. *A Medicare Voucher System: What Can It Offer?* Presented to the Conference on the Future of Medicare, sponsored by the Committee on Ways and Means, the Congressional Budget Office and the Congressional Research Service, November 29–30.

Friedman, E., 1984. Medi-Cal Contracting: Model or Mayhem? *Hospitals* 58 (1):74–78.

Gabel, J., and D. Ermann. 1985. Preferred Provider Organizations: Performance, Problems, and Promise. *Health Affairs* 4 (1):24–40.

Garfinkel, S. A., W. E. Schlesinger, K. R. McLeroy et al. 1986. Choice of Payment Plan in the Medicare Capitation Demonstration. *Medical Care* 24 (7):628–40.

Ginsburg, P. B. 1983. Market-Oriented Options in Medicare and Medicaid. In *Market Reforms in Health Care: Current Issues, New Directions, Strategic Decisions*, ed. J. A. Meyer, pp. 103–17. Washington: American Enterprise Institute for Public Policy Research.

Goldberg, V. 1975. Some Emerging Problems of Prepaid Health Plans in the Medi-Cal System. *Policy Analysis* 1(Winter):55–68.

Goldsmith, J. 1984. Death of a Paradigm: The Challenge of Competition. *Health Affairs* 3 (3):5–19.

Greenberg, W. 1983. How Will Increased Competition Affect the Costs of Health Care? In *Market Reforms in Health Care: Current Issues, New Directions, Strategic Decisions*, ed. J. A. Meyer, pp. 46–60. Washington: American Enterprise Institute for Public Policy Research.

Greenfield, C. A. 1986. Improving Elderly Access to Health Care Information. *Business and Health* 3 (7):26–30.

Greenlick, M., S. Lamb, T. Carpenter et al. 1983. Kaiser-Permanente's Medicare Plus Project: A Successful Medicare Prospective Payment Demonstration. *Health Care Financing Review* 4 (4):85–97.

Gruenberg, L., S. Wallack and C. Tomkins. 1986. Pricing Strategies for Capitated Delivery Systems. *Health Care Financing Review* (Annual Supplement):35–44.

Hagen, R. 1986. Medigap Insurance: Pitfalls and Progress. *Business and Health* 3 (5):25–30.

Havighurst, C. C. 1983. Decentralizing Decision Making: Private Contract Versus Professional Norms. In *Market Reforms in Health Care: Current Issues, New Directions, Strategic Decisions*, ed. J. A. Meyer, pp. 22–45. Washington: American Enterprise Institute for Public Policy Research.

Hirschman, A. 1970. *Exit, Voice, and Loyalty*. Cambridge: Harvard University Press.

Holmes, D., M. Shadle, J. McGee et al. 1986. *National HMO Firm: 1985*. Excelsior, MN: Interstudy.

Hospital Week. 1986. GAO Report Calls for Cuts in Capitated Rates. *Hospital Week* 22 (27):1–20.

Iglehart, J. K. 1985a. Congress, Public Policy, and the Future: A Conversation with Bill Gradison. *Health Affairs* 4 (4):41–49.

———. 1985b. Medicare Turns to HMOs. *New England Journal of Medicine* 312 (2):132–37.

Interstudy. 1985. *National HMO Census: 1985*. Excelsior, MN.

Iversen, L. H., and C. L. Polich. 1985. *The Future of Medicare and HMOs*. Excelsior, MN: Interstudy.

Iversen, L. H., C. L. Polich and J. R. Dahl. 1985. *The 1985 Medicare and HMOs Data Book*. Excelsior, MN: Interstudy.

Kerschner, P. A. 1986. Are DRGs Affecting Just the Elderly? *Business and Health* 3 (5): 31–37.

Langwell, K. and J. Hadley. 1986. Capitation and the Medicare Program: History, Issues and Evidence. *Health Care Financing Review* Annual Supplement: 9–20.

LaTour, S. A., B. Friedman and E. F. X. Hughes. 1986. Medicare Beneficiary Decision Making About Health Insurance: Implications for a Voucher System. *Medical Care* 24 (7):601–13.

Leutz, W., J. Greenberg, R. Abrahams et al., 1985. *Changing Health Care For An Aging Society*. Lexington, MA: Lexington Books.

Lissovoy, G., T. Rice, D. Ermann et al. 1986. Preferred Provider Organizations: Today's Models and Tomorrow's Prospects. *Inquiry* 23 (1):7–15.

Luft, H. S. 1981. *Health Maintenance Organizations: Dimensions of Performance*. New York: Wiley.

———. 1982. Health Maintenance Organizations and the Rationing of Medical Care. *Milbank Memorial Fund Quarterly* 60 (2):268–306.

McCall, N., T. Rice and J. Sangl. 1986. Consumer Knowledge of Medicare and Supplemental Health Insurance Benefits. *Health Service Research* 20 (6):633–57.

McClure, W. 1984. On the Research Status of Risk-Adjusted Capitation Rates. *Inquiry* 21(Fall):205–13.

Manning, W. G., A. Leibowitz, G. A. Goldberg et al. 1984. A Controlled Trial of the Effect of a Prepaid Group Practice on Use of Services. *New England Journal of Medicine* 310 (23):1505–10.

Manton, K., and K. Liu. 1984. *The Future Growth of the Long-Term Care Population: Projections Based on the 1977 National Nursing Home Survey and the 1982 Long-Term-Care Survey*. Paper presented at the Third National Leadership Conference on Long-Term Care Issues, Washington, March 7–9.

Meier, G., and J. Tillotson. 1978. *Physician Reimbursement and Hospital Use in HMOs*. Excelsior, MN: Interstudy.

W. M. Mercer–Meidinger, Inc. 1986. *Trends and Influences in Corporate Mental Health Programs*. A Report to the American Psychiatric Association. May.

Pollack, W. 1979. *Expanding Health Benefits for the Elderly*, Volume 1, *Long-term Care*. Washington: Urban Institute Press.

Rice, T., G. de Lissovoy, J. Gabel et al. 1985. The State of PPOs: Results from a National Survey. *Health Affairs* 4 (4):25–40.

Rich, S. 1986. Chrysler Proposes Medicare Role. *Washington Post*. April 8:1.

Rossiter, L., A. Friedlob and K. Langwell. 1985. Exploring Benefits of Risk-Based Contracting Under Medicare. *Health Care Financial Management* 39 (5):42–57.

Rowe, J. W. 1985. Health Care of the Elderly. *New England Journal of Medicine* 312 (13):827–35.

Ruchlin, H. J. Morris and G. Eggert. 1982. Management and Financing of Long-Term Care Services: A New Approach to a Chronic Problem. *New England Journal of Medicine* 306 (2):101–5.

Sapolsky, H. 1977. America's Socialized Medicine: The Allocation of Resources Within the Veterans' Health Care System. *Public Policy* 25 (3):359–82.

Schlesinger, M. 1986. On the Limits of Expanding Health Care Reform: Chronic Care in Prepaid Settings. *Milbank Quarterly* 64 (2);189–215.

Schlesinger, M., D. Blumenthal and E. Schlesinger. 1986. Profits Under Pressure: The Economic Performance of Investor-Owned and Nonprofit Health Maintenance Organizations. *Medical Care* 24 (7):615–27.

Sloan, F. A. and E. R. Becker. 1984. Cross-subsidies and Payment for Hospital Care. *Journal of Health Politics, Policy and Law* 8 (4):660–85.

Somers, A. 1984. Why Not Try Preventing Illness as a Way of Controling Medicare Costs? *New England Journal of Medicine* 311 (13):853–56.

Sorian, R. 1986. Florida HMO's Problems Continue. *Medicine and Health* 40 (17):1.

Sullivan, S., and P. W. Samors. 1983. Administrative Proposals for Health Care Reform. In *Market Reforms in Health Care: Current Issues, New Directions, Strategic Decisions*, ed. J. A. Meyer, pp. 225–40. Washington: American Enterprise Institute for Public Policy Research.

Taylor, H., and M. Kagay. 1986. The HMO Report Card: A Closer Look. *Health Affairs* 5 (1):81–89.

Thomas, J. W., and R. Lichtenstein. 1986. Functional Health Measure for Adjusting Health

Maintenance Organization Capitation Rates. *Health Care Financing Review* 7 (3):85–95.

Traska, M. R. 1986. Former Risk Contractors Are Leery of Rule Changes. *Hospitals* 60 (13):82.

U.S. Congress, Office of Technology Assessment. 1986. *Payment for Physicians' Services: Strategies for Medicare*. Publication No. OTA-H-294. Washington, D.C.: U.S. Government Printing Office.

Verway, V. A. 1985. New Uses of Copayments by HMOs: Regulatory Considerations. *HMOs Confronting New Challenges, June 1985*. Conference Proceedings, Annual Meeting of Group Health Association of America, pp.

Ware, J., W. Rogers, A. Davies et al. 1986. Comparison of Health Outcomes at a Health Maintenance Organization with Those in Fee-for-Service Care. *Lancet* 16(May 3):1017–22.

Well, P. 1976. Comparative Costs to the Medicare Program of Seven Prepaid Group Practices and Controls. *Milbank Memorial Fund Quarterly* 54 (3):339–60.

Wilensky, G. R., and L. F. Rossiter. 1986. Patient Self-Selection in HMOs. *Health Affairs* 5 (2):66–80.

Winn, S. and K. McCaffree, 1979. Issues Involved in the Development of a Prepaid Capitation Plan for Long-term Care Services. *Gerontologist* 19 (3):184–90.

Yelin, E. H., C. J. Henke, J. S. Kramer et al. 1985. A Comparison of the Treatment of Rheumatoid Arthritis in Health Maintenance Organizations and Fee-for-Service Practices. *New England Journal of Medicine* 312 (15):962–67.

8

Medicare Financing: The Government's Share

NANCY J. ALTMAN
ALICIA H. MUNNELL
JAMES M. VERDIER

Medicare is financed through two trust funds: the Hospital Insurance (HI) trust fund covers Part A of the program, and the Supplementary Medical Insurance (SMI) trust fund finances Part B. The funds are operated on a pay-as-you-go basis, which means that revenues are disbursed for program expenses as soon as they are collected.

Both funds are projected to face financing problems in the future. The most recent projections for the HI trust fund show that resources may be depleted by 2002. Similarly, the required contribution to SMI from general revenues is expected to grow faster than the government's tax receipts.

Medicare's financing problems should not be solved simply by raising more money because promising opportunities for cost control exist and should be pursued. However, the prospect of insolvency in the HI trust fund and the strain on general revenues from the SMI trust fund require policymakers to survey the options for increasing Medicare revenues while cost-control devices are being developed. Indeed, even if cost-control efforts were completely successful, additional revenues would be needed to finance new initiatives in the Medicare program.

This chapter will first review the financial status of the Medicare trust funds. Then it will examine a variety of options for increasing revenues.

Outlook for the Medicare Trust Funds

Uncertainty surrounding (1) the effectiveness of cost-control measures and (2) future economic and demographic trends makes projecting Medicare outlays an extremely difficult exercise. Each year, the Board of Trustees of the HI and SMI trust funds prepares four alternative forecasts of income and expenditures under differing sets of assumptions. Alternatives II-A and II-B represent intermediate cost increase assumptions. Alternative I is based on more optimistic, lower-cost assumptions. Alternative III involves pessimistic assumptions.[1]

Outlook for the HI Fund

Revenues for the HI program are primarily derived from the Social Security payroll tax. In 1987, the HI payroll-tax rate was 1.45 percent each for the employee and the employer on earnings up to the taxable maximum of $43,800. The tax rate is scheduled to remain at 1.45 percent for future years, but the maximum taxable earnings limit will rise automatically each year to reflect growth in average wages.

The balances in the HI trust fund increased steadily from 1966, the first year benefits were paid, through 1981, when the HI fund held $19 billion, an amount equal to 61 percent of annual outlays (Table 8–1). However, substantial borrowing by the Old Age and Survivors Insurance (OASI) trust fund in 1982 reduced HI balances to $13 billion in 1983. A lump-sum general revenue transfer brought balances in 1984 to $16 billion, and increases in the combined tax rate from 2.6 percent to 2.9 percent, along with a higher level of earnings in covered employment, helped restore the HI fund balances to $40 billion in 1986.[2]

The 1987 Trustees Report projects that annual surpluses for the next eight years will allow the trust fund balance to increase through 1994. Beyond that year, annual deficits are expected gradually to reduce accumulated reserves, until the fund is depleted in 2002. The most pessimistic projection indicates that insolvency could occur six years earlier.

The surpluses are a result of two special factors. First, the OASI trust fund repaid a large portion of its loan to the HI fund in 1986, and second, the HI payroll tax increased by about 12 percent from 1984 to 1986.[3] Now that the tax increases have taken effect and the OASI loans are repaid, income growth should taper off and average about 6 percent over the next 10 years.

Estimates of changes in the basic cost of providing hospital care are derived from a market basket of goods and services purchased by hospitals. The labor costs in this basket are projected to increase by roughly 5 percent per year over the next decade while capital costs are scheduled to rise 4.5 percent on average. These increases, along with a 0.25 percent additional increase to allow for improvements in medical technology, are assumed for purposes of adjusting the diagnostic-related-group (DRG) rates under the new prospective payment system.

Additional annual increases in HI outlays stem from (1) increases in program enrollment, projected to average nearly 1.5 percent per year over the next 14 years and (2) hospital admission rates, which, after a decline of slightly more than 3 percent over 1986, are scheduled to increase at an annual rate of 1 to 2 percent until 2000. Finally, the Trustees' projections include an increase of nearly 1 percent a year to allow for miscellaneous uncontrolled expenses (such as a shift toward higher-cost admissions). These three factors plus the increase in DRG rates yield an average outlay growth of over 8 percent per year from 1986 to 2000.

A glance at a series of projections for the HI trust fund by the Board of Trustees shows that the outlook has improved in recent years (Figure 8–1). Most of the improvement between the 1983–84 forecasts and those of 1985–86 is due to lower projected outlay growth. For example, in 1984, predicted 1985 outlays were $4.3 billion higher than actual outlays, an excess of almost 9 percent. The cumulative effect of the real 1985 outlays was that the HI exhaustion date was extended almost five years.

TABLE 8–1 Past and Projected Operations of the HI Trust Fund,[a] Selected Calendar Years, 1966–2002 ($ billions)

Year	*Income*	*Outlays*	*Net Increase in Fund*[b]	*Fund at End of Year*
1966	$ 2	$ 1	$ 1	$ 1
1970	6	5	1	3
1975	13	12	1	11
1980	26	26	1	14
1981	36	31	5	19
1982	38	36	−11	8
1983	45	40	5	13
1984	47	44	3	16
1985	51	48	5	21
1986	59	50	19	40
1987	63	49	14	54
1988	67	56	11	66
1989	72	62	10	76
1990	77	68	9	85
1991	83	75	7	92
1992	88	83	6	98
1993	94	90	4	102
1994	99	98	1	103
1995	105	107	−2	101
1996	111	115	−5	97
1997	117	124	−8	89
1998	123	134	−11	78
1999	129	145	−16	62
2000	136	156	−21	41
2001	143	169	−26	15
2002	149	181	−32	[c]

[a]Projections are from Alternative II-B of the Board of Trustees 1987 Report.

[b]Net increase in fund includes transfers of assets among the Old Age and Survivors Insurance (OASI), Disability Insurance (DI), and Hospital Insurance (HI) trust funds under the interfund borrowing authority provided by PL 97–123. These transfers include $12.4 billion borrowed by OASI from HI in 1982 and a $1.8 billion repayment of this loan in 1985 with the remaining $10.6 billion repaid in 1986.

[c]Fund depleted in 2002.

Source: Social Security Administration, 1987a. Table 6, p. 40; Table 11, p. 53.

The slowdown in growth of outlays may be due in part to the introduction of the new prospective payment system (PPS) which pays hospitals a predetermined rate per admission based on DRGs. However, separating the transitional from the permanent effects of this system is not yet possible. Although most observers expected hospital admissions to increase for those age 65 and over, the introduction of PPS has actually been accompanied by a dip in the rate of increase of these

FIGURE. 8–1 HI-Trust Fund Projections, Alternative Views

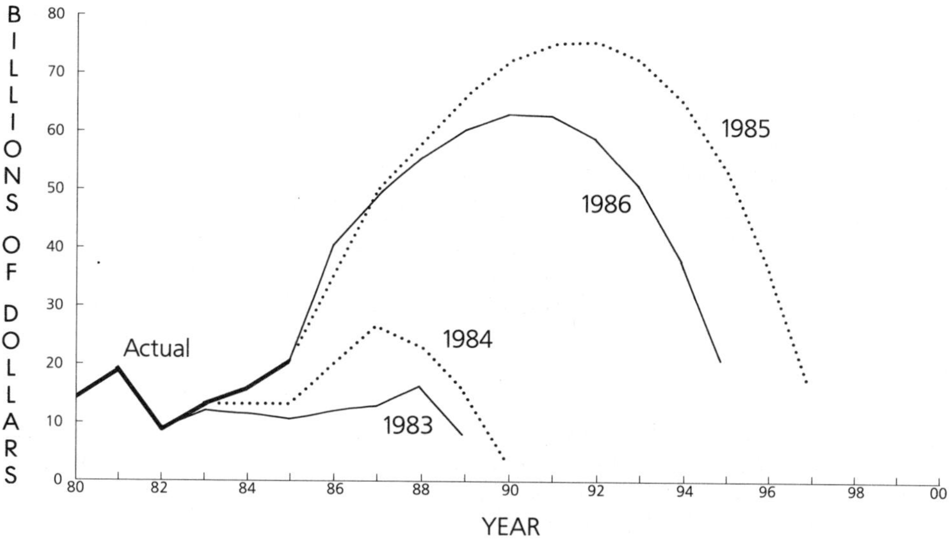

Sources: 1986 Annual Report of the Board of Trustees of the Federal Hospital Insurance Trust Fund, Table 6, p. 35, and Table 11, p. 48; 1985 Annual Report of the Board of Trustees of the Federal Hospital Insurance Trust Fund, Table 10, p. 42; 1984 Annual Report of the Board of Trustees of the Federal Hospital Insurance Trust Fund, Table 10, p. 36; 1983 Annual Report of the Board of Trustees of the Federal Hospital Insurance Trust Fund, Table 10, p. 46.

admissions. Temporary adjustment problems might reduce HI outlays in the short run but would not be expected to affect the long-run level of activity. The reaction of hospitals to the new payment system remains a major uncertainty surrounding projections of future HI outlays.

Many experts doubt that the DRG system will be an effective cost control mechanism without corresponding control on admissions and other adjustments (see Chapter 5). However, other approaches, such as encouraging the growth of health maintenance organizations (HMOs) and state and local government cost-control plans may have a more enduring effect on hospital costs.

Further questions exist regarding DRG rate increases after 1987 because no limits are specified in the current law. Instead, annual changes in DRG rates will be determined by the secretary of Health and Human Services (DHHS) in consultation with a newly established Prospective Payment Assessment Commission. As discussed earlier, HI trustees assume that increases in DRG rates will be equal to increases in the price of the market basket of hospital services plus 0.25 percent. Modifying the baseline assumption by a one-percentage-point increase or decrease in the rate of change for Medicare hospital reimbursement would have a substantial impact on the projected date for trust fund insolvency.

In short, considerable uncertainty over the financial future of the HI trust fund exists. Alternative I indicates that the fund could remain solvent over the next 25 years. However, all other Trustees' forecasts indicate a future imbalance between outlays and income as a result of soaring hospital costs.

Outlook for the SMI Fund

SMI revenues come from (1) premiums paid by participants and (2) general revenues.[4] During 1987 the premium was $17.90 per month, which was designed to produce income equal to 25 percent of program costs.[5] The difference between premium income and annual SMI outlays is made up by general revenues. For 1987, general revenue contributions to SMI are estimated at $20 billion.

Although appropriations from general revenues must, by law, be sufficient to guarantee the solvency of the SMI trust fund, the financial demands of this program remain a source of concern. Disbursements under SMI are projected to grow at an average of 16 percent per year over the next three years (Table 8–2). While no long-run projections are made for this program, the rapid growth in disbursements is unlikely to decrease in the future. Although the SMI trust fund is not faced with insolvency in the conventional sense, its financial requirements are an important component of the outlook for Medicare.

The most recent projections for Medicare reveal that additional money will be needed to maintain current benefit levels if cost-control efforts do not reduce the rate of growth of outlays. Even if costs were brought under control, additional revenues would be necessary if the program were expanded to cover catastrophic insurance, prescription drugs and additional long-term care benefits. Therefore, the following sections will examine possible sources of revenues for financing Medicare.

Possible Sources of Federal Revenues for Medicare Financing

The federal government's major revenue source is a progressive tax on the incomes of individuals. The personal income tax, which is administered primarily by withholding a portion of wages as they are earned, generated approximately $360 billion in fiscal year 1987.

The federal government's second largest revenue source is the payroll tax, used to finance the HI component of Medicare and the cash-benefit programs of Social Security. Payroll taxes accounted for approximately $300 billion in revenues in 1987. Receipts from revenue sources currently used by the federal government are displayed in Table 8–3.

An important concern in evaluating Medicare revenue sources is the appropriate distribution of the financing burden. Arguably, the current distribution embodies an implicit political consensus on the proper allocation of the financing burden: workers cover roughly 50 percent of total HI and SMI costs by way of the payroll tax, beneficiaries about 25 percent through premiums and cost sharing, and taxpayers about 20 percent through general revenues. Approximately 5 percent comes from interest on the trust funds' assets (Table 8–4).

However, appropriate sources of *additional* revenue are subject to debate. One consideration is the available tax base. Table 8–5 shows the incomes of people younger than 65 and those 65 and over by income class and income source. In 1984, the 87 million taxpayers under 65 received more than 90 percent of their income from wages and salaries, while the 12 million taxpayers 65 and over received nearly 80 percent of their income from investments. Indeed, the $191 billion in investment

TABLE 8–2 Past and Projected Operations of the SMI Trust Fund, Selected Calendar Years, 1966–93 ($ billions)[a]

Year	*Income*	*Outlays*	*Net Increase in Fund*	*Fund at End of Year*
1966	$ b	$ b	$ b	$ b
1970	2	2	b	b
1975	5	5	b	1
1980	11	11	b	5
1981	15	14	1	6
1982	17	16	b	6
1983	20	19	1	7
1984	23	21	3	10
1985	25	24	1	11
1986	25	27	−2	8
1987	28	32	−4	5
1988	38	36	2	6
1989	43	42	1	8
1990	49	48	1	9
1991	56	55	1	10
1992	64	63	1	11
1993	73	72	1	12

[a]Totals may not add owing to rounding.
[b]less than $0.5 billion.
Source: Social Security Administration, 1987b. Table 6, p. 30.

income received by those 65 and over exceeded the $166 billion in investment income received by all other taxpayers.

The amount of additional revenue necessary to fund Medicare is another important consideration when choosing revenue sources. Obviously, collection mechanisms already in place are less expensive than those requiring new or substantially modified procedures. However, insufficiently considered increases in current taxes could have adverse economic consequences. For example, raising the payroll tax might prompt employers to lower wages.

The final and perhaps most important factor when judging financing sources is political acceptability. Largely based on public perceptions that are imperfectly informed and subject to change, political acceptability is difficult to assess. However,

TABLE 8–3 Sources of Governmental Revenue, Fiscal Year 1987 ($ billions)

Individual income taxes	$361
Corporate income taxes	100
Payroll taxes	301
Excise taxes	33
Other	39
Total	834

Source: U.S. Congressional Budget Office. February 1987.

TABLE 8-4 Distribution of Medicare Financing Burden, Years 1968–84: Spending on and by Aged Beneficiaries (percentage of program costs)

Year[a]	*Beneficiary*	*Payroll Tax*	*General Federal Revenues*	*Other*[b]
1968	28%	56%	10%	6%
1969	25	52	12	11
1970	20	59	11	10
1971	28	49	12	11
1972	29	50	13	8
1973	27	58	9	6
1974	24	61	9	6
1975	25	59	9	7
1976	25	58	9	8
1977	24	50	19	7
1978	23	53	17	7
1979	24	55	15	6
1980	24	55	15	6
1981	21	57	17	5
1982	26	52	16	6
1983	22	50	17	11
1984	23	52	18	7

[a]Fiscal years 1968–76; calendar years 1977–84.

[b]Interest, transfers from railroad retirement account, payments for military wage credits and reimbursement for uninsured persons.

TABLE 8-5 Income of Taxpayers Under Age 65 and 65 and Over (1984 income tax returns)[a b]

	Under Age 65			*Age 65 and Over*		
Adjusted Gross Income	*Number of Returns (millions)*	*Wage and Salary Income ($ billions)*	*Investment Income*[c] *($ billions)*	*Number of Returns (millions)*	*Wage and Salary Income ($ billions)*	*Investment Income*[c] *($ billions)*
$0–10,000	29	$ 136	$ 17	4	$ 6	$ 22
$10–20,000	22	295	20	4	11	46
$20–30,000	15	348	20	2	9	28
$30–50,000	16	574	33	1	13	33
$50–100,000	5	289	31	1	9	29
$100,000 or more	1	108	46	d	10	32
	88	1,750	166	12	58	191

[a]Details may not add to totals owing to rounding.

[b]Although the data in Table 8-5 show only income reported on tax returns and only about 60 percent of those 65 and over file tax returns, almost all of those who do not file have very low incomes.

[c]Includes interest, capital gains, pensions, annuities, dividends, rents, royalties, estates and trusts.

[d]Less than 0.5 million.

Source: Adapted from Internal Revenue Service, *Individual Income Tax Returns 1984* (Pub. 1304 [11-86]). Tables 1.4 and 2.5.

one important determinant of public support of Medicare is its resemblance to private insurance.

This resemblance is quite close for HI, where the revenue to pay benefits (other than interest income) comes only from current or future potential beneficiaries. While nearly three-fourths of the financing for SMI comes from general revenues, it is less visible to the public than the 25 percent from beneficiary premiums and cost sharing. The resemblance to private insurance is further enhanced by labeling the payroll taxes for Medicare as contributions and segregating the income into separate trust funds. Like private insurance, eligibility depends on payment of contributions or premiums.

More fundamentally, Medicare, like private insurance, pools risk. Unsubsidized risk pooling is quite straightforward: If 10 people know that 1 of them will suffer a $50 loss, all may choose to contribute $5 in order to offset their own possible losses. Many forms of insurance also supply subsidies for certain members of the pool. Unisex mortality tables, for example, result in men subsidizing women in the purchase of annuities, and women subsidizing men in the purchase of life insurance. Similarly, when experience is not taken into account in setting insurance rates, healthier people subsidize the less healthy.

Medicare contains a variety of subsidies not found in private insurance. For example, those with higher lifetime-covered wages subsidize those with lower lifetime-covered wages. That is, contributions to HI vary with wages earned up to the taxable wage limit, while coverage is identical. Medicare also includes subsidies of earlier generations by later ones. This is a result of the pay-as-you-go nature of Medicare financing, the increasing costs of medical care, the decision to cover the initial beneficiaries without requiring payment of taxes and the variance in the size of different age groups. Additionally, the program subsidizes nonworking spouses of beneficiaries by those who are unmarried or have working spouses. Because of these additional subsidies, Medicare is often referred to as *social* insurance.

If retaining the perception of Medicare as an insurance program is important to its continued public support, financing proposals should be judged at least in part by the extent to which they reaffirm that perception. Financing proposals that break the perceived link between payments and benefits or erode the image of Medicare as an insurance program could threaten its political acceptability.

Options for Financing Medicare

In the following discussion, options for raising Medicare revenue are divided into taxes on workers, taxes on beneficiaries and taxes on the general population. Table 8-6 summarizes the options.[6]

Taxes on Workers

Currently about 85 percent of the HI Fund's income is from payroll taxes. The payroll tax contains no exemptions or deductions, and taxes are levied only on wages at or below the maximum taxable wage base and do not apply to investment income.

TABLE 8-6 Medicare Financing Options and Estimated Revenue Gain, Fiscal Year 1991 ($ billions)

Options	*Revenue Gain Fiscal Year 1991*
Increase Medicare payroll tax by 0.5 percentage points	$13
Apply Medicare payroll tax to all earnings	8
Extend Medicare payroll taxes to all state and local workers	2
Apply Medicare payroll tax to all employee fringe benefits	13
Impose income tax on insurance value of Medicare benefits	6
Impose 30 percent tax on Medigap premiums	6
Eliminate higher income tax standard deduction for the elderly	2
Impose 1 percent individual income tax surcharge	5
Impose 1 percent corporate income tax surcharge	1
Double federal excise taxes on alcohol	6
Increase cigarette excise tax to $0.32 per pack	5

Sources: Munnell, 1985, pp. 46–61; U.S. Congressional Budget Office (March 1986); U.S. Congressional Budget Office, January 1987; and authors' estimates.

While these tax features are regressive, they enhance the resemblance of Medicare to a private insurance system, adding to its political acceptability and stability.

Among the most viable means of increasing Medicare revenues through payroll taxes are increasing the existing payroll tax rate, including all state and local government workers in the taxable population, broadening the payroll tax base to include noncash benefits and reallocating revenues from the Social Security cash-benefit programs (OASDI) to Medicare.

RAISE PAYROLL TAX RATE

Increasing the payroll tax rate is the simplest and most straightforward option. The mechanism for collecting the tax is already in place, and its broad base assures that large amounts of money can be raised without dramatically increasing the burden on any single worker. A 0.5 percentage point increase—to 1.95 percent each on employers and employees—would raise about $13 billion in fiscal year 1991, (U.S. Congressional Budget Office, 1986), but the largest yearly increase for any worker would only be $219 at 1987 income levels (.5% × $43,800).

The burden of an increase in payroll taxes on lower-income workers could be offset for lower-income workers by increasing the earned income tax credit. This credit, as modified by the Tax Reform Act of 1986, allows workers with children an income tax credit or direct payment equal to 14 percent of their first $5,714 of wage and salary income. It is phased out for incomes over $9,000, dropping to zero at $17,000. An increase in the earned income tax credit to 14.5 percent would entirely offset the direct impact of a 0.5-percent payroll tax increase for incomes under $9,000, and partially offset it for incomes between $9,000 and $17,000.

INCREASE PAYROLL TAX BASE

A more progressive option is raising the level of earnings subject to the payroll tax. Currently, approximately 90 percent of total earnings are subject to the payroll tax. The most extreme version of this approach—entirely removing the tax cap for both employers and employees—would generate about $41 billion in additional revenue in 1991, $8 billion of which would go to the HI trust fund. However, this method would simultaneously increase the benefits owed by the cash programs of Social Security because they are based on the level of covered wages paid. Less-extreme versions might limit the increase to just the HI portion of the payroll tax or maintain the wage cap for the employees' share of the tax. However, increasing only the HI portion of the tax is administratively difficult, and increasing just the employers' share politically unlikely; the parity between employer and employee taxes results in some fiscal constraint on the program thereby helping to maintain business support. A 1977 Carter administration proposal to lift the wage cap for employers was defeated because of substantial business opposition.

EXTEND MEDICARE PAYROLL TAXES TO ALL STATE AND LOCAL GOVERNMENT WORKERS

About 20 percent of state and local government employees do not pay Medicare payroll taxes, although most of these workers qualify for Medicare benefits as a result of earlier or subsequent nongovernmental employment. Consequently, they receive the same benefits as other workers but do not pay as much into the system. In 1985 Congress extended contribution liability to all state and local employees hired after March 31, 1986 (Consolidated Omnibus Budget Reconciliation Act of 1985), but employees hired before that date continue to receive windfall benefits.

Requiring all currently uncovered state and local workers and their employers to pay Medicare payroll taxes would raise about $2 billion in 1991.

BROADEN PAYROLL TAX BASE TO INCLUDE FRINGE BENEFITS

At present, employer contributions to qualified employee pensions, group health insurance and group life insurance are not taxed as income to the employee under either the income tax or the payroll tax. Between 1950 and 1984, these benefits have increased from 2.6 to 10.4 percent of total compensation, significantly eroding both the income-tax and the payroll-tax bases and raising the tax rates required to finance the Social Security system over the long run (Munnell, 1985).

Excluding the value of fringe benefits has also created inequities in the tax system. First, two individuals who are equally well-off in an economic sense will pay different amounts of payroll and income taxes over their lifetimes. Second, such an exclusion has an adverse impact on income distribution because fringe benefits are concentrated among higher-paid employees, while all taxpayers pay higher taxes to compensate for the favorable tax treatment accorded employee benefits.

Subjecting noncash benefits to the HI payroll tax would raise about $13 billion in 1991 and make the payroll tax more progressive because a larger share of the burden would fall on highly paid workers who have more generous fringe benefits.

There have been several proposals to include noncash benefits in taxable income. Both the Treasury Department in 1984 and President Reagan in 1985 proposed including a portion of employer-paid health insurance premiums in employees' taxable income for both income-tax and payroll-tax purposes. However, the administrative difficulties in valuing these benefits and collecting taxes on them are significant enough to discourage setting up an administrative apparatus solely to collect Medicare payroll taxes. Therefore, this option is most feasible in the context of broader tax reform, where fringe benefits could be subjected in comparable fashion to both income and payroll taxes.

Reallocate Existing Payroll Taxes

The projected deficits in the Medicare trust funds are expected to coincide with substantial annual surpluses in the OASDI program. An alternative to raising new revenue is to reallocate a portion of the scheduled OASDI tax receipts to Medicare.

The OASDI trust funds are expected to produce surpluses in the range of $50 billion to $200 billion a year during the 1990s—between 1 and 2 percent of projected gross national product (Social Security Administration, 1986). These surpluses are the result of payroll-tax increases and benefit reductions enacted in 1977 and 1983. Reserves are projected to build up over the next 35 years and they will then be used to cover deficits created when the baby-boom generation reaches retirement age. Under this system, the baby-boom generation will be the first to prepay a large share of its retirement benefits during its working years. Previous generations have benefited from Social Security's pay-as-you-go system, in which the current generation of workers pays for the benefits of the current generation of retirees, with no buildup in the trust fund beyond a small contingency reserve.

The existence of a large pool of reserve assets should help to ensure that future benefit commitments are fulfilled without raising tax rates in the years after 2020. Nevertheless, it is worthwhile to consider the possibility of a contribution from OASDI reserves into the HI trust fund. Precedents exist for the transfer of revenues from one fund to another. In 1982 the OASDI trust funds were able to finance operations during a temporary shortage of funds by borrowing from the HI trust fund. Unfortunately, the projections discussed earlier suggest that HI's problem is more than a temporary one.

A permanent transfer of funds to HI from OASDI raises the broader question of whether the OASDI fund buildup should be preserved intact and, if not, whether HI's claim on some portion of it is strong enough to justify a transfer.

The large projected buildup in OASDI funds could have a detrimental effect on the economy. Projections under current law put the OASDI surplus at roughly $10 trillion by 2020—more than 28 percent of projected GNP in that year (Munnell and Blais, 1984). At the very least, it may be difficult for the economy to adjust to this degree of forced saving.

Once this surplus begins to accumulate, proposals will undoubtedly be made to use it for purposes other than prefunding the retirement costs of the baby-boom generation. Possibilities range from reductions in Social Security payroll taxes and increases in benefits to reductions in other taxes or increases in other forms of spending.

Using part of the OASDI surplus to finance deficits in the HI trust fund is more closely related to the purposes of the OASDI trust funds than many other possible uses. Nonetheless, such a reallocation raises questions of intergenerational equity that should be directly addressed. In effect, the fund that is being set aside to pay

Social Security retirement benefits to the baby-boom generation would be used instead to pay Medicare benefits to the current generation of retirees.

If this reallocation approach were adopted, the OASDI trust fund would experience a shortfall after 2020. A probable solution is an increase in payroll taxes for the post-2020 generation of workers—the children of the baby boomers. Current estimates suggest that an increase of a little more than one percentage point each for employers and employees would be sufficient (Munnell, 1985). The baby-boom generation would thus have a larger share of their retirement costs paid for by their children to make up for their paying a greater share of the costs of retirees in the 1990s—a partial return to pay-as-you-go financing.

The major alternatives to using part of the OASDI surplus to finance projected Medicare deficits are (1) to increase payroll taxes on the current generation of workers or (2) to reduce benefits for the current generation of retirees. The costs of these options are clear and immediate, while the costs of dipping into the OASDI surplus will only occur some 30 years from now, when payroll taxes may have to be increased or benefits reduced.

There is one potential cost, however, that is more immediate, if less tangible. The confidence of the current generation of workers that Social Security will be able to pay them the retirement benefits they are being promised—shaken by recent bankruptcy scares—could be eroded further if the OASDI funds are drawn down. This could reduce support for Social Security among a large and important segment of the public.[7]

Taxes on Beneficiaries

As noted earlier, beneficiaries now pay slightly less than 25 percent of the cost of Medicare through SMI premiums and copayments, deductibles and liability for unassigned physicians' charges in HI and SMI. Beneficiary financing of this kind is consistent with insurance principles, but it can place a substantial burden on lower-income beneficiaries. A variety of proposals for modifying beneficiary financing are discussed in Chapter 3. Three additional proposals are discussed here because in part they potentially involve use of the income tax system.

Income Tax on Insurance Value of Medicare Benefits

If health insurance benefits provided by private employers were subject to the income tax, as proposed by President Reagan among others, a logical step would be to tax the insurance value of Medicare (not the benefits paid out) in the same way. A tax on the employer and government-provided shares of HI and SMI would increase income tax revenues by about $6 billion a year in 1991 (U.S. Congressional Budget Office, 1987a). Following the precedent of the Social Security Act amendments of 1983 that assigned the income taxes collected on Social Security benefits to the OASDI trust funds, the income taxes collected on Medicare benefits could be earmarked for Medicare.

Because elderly with low incomes do not pay any income tax, they would be unaffected by this proposal. Elderly beneficiaries with higher incomes, however, could face additional income taxes of nearly $500 per year (U.S. Congressional Budget Office, 1987). To ease this burden, the same threshold that applies to taxation of Social Security benefits could be used: Individuals with incomes up to

$25,000 and couples with incomes up to $32,000 would be exempt from extra tax. This formula would generate a revenue gain of about $4 billion in 1991.

Tax on Medigap Policies

Nearly 70 percent of the participants in Medicare also have Medigap policies, which primarily cover the cost-sharing portions of Medicare. By reducing beneficiaries' incentives to economize on the use of services, these policies increase the overall costs of the Medicare program. A 30 percent tax on Medigap premiums would raise roughly $6 billion in 1991, simultaneously offsetting some of these additional Medicare costs and reducing the incentive to purchase Medigap policies. The proceeds of this tax could be added to the Medicare trust funds.

Unfortunately, administration of a Medigap tax would be complicated. Only about 50 percent of the elderly file income tax returns, making the income tax an ineffective collection mechanism. An excise tax on the policies, which required the sellers to collect the tax and remit it to the government, would be more practical. If the tax were stated separately on policyholders' bills, beneficiaries would be aware of the added cost.

Elimination of Extra Standard Deduction for the Elderly

The Tax Reform Act of 1986 allows an extra standard deduction of $600 ($750 if not married) for those over 65 and the blind. (This provision takes the place of the extra personal exemption for the elderly and the blind under prior law.) Eliminating this extra standard deduction for the elderly would increase income tax revenues by about $2 billion in fiscal year 1991. This extra income tax revenue could be assigned to the Medicare trust funds and thus function as a kind of indirect income-tested premium.[8] The low-income elderly would would not be affected at all, since they pay no income taxes, while those with higher incomes would pay progressively higher amounts. The extra $600 standard deduction saves a person in the 15 percent bracket $90 in taxes, while someone in the top 28 percent bracket saves $168.

Taxes on the General Population

About 70 percent of the SMI program and 20 percent of total Medicare costs are currently covered from general revenues. General revenue financing is more progressive than the Medicare payroll tax because roughly 70 percent of general revenues come from the personal income tax and another 15 percent from the corporate income tax.[9]

The link between Social Security benefits and lifetime wages makes the payroll tax a logical financing source for the OASDI trust funds. Under Medicare, by contrast, health benefits do not vary according to previous earnings, so general revenue financing is easier to justify. Indeed, general revenues have always played a significant role in financing Medicare through the SMI portion of the program.

The issue is whether the relative contribution from general revenues should increase. General revenue financing is not consistent with the insurance principle, which encourages financing solely through beneficiaries. Increasing it might thus erode some of the political support that Medicare now has. While general revenue financing of part of SMI has not noticeably reduced the political support for that program, this aspect of SMI's financing is not highly visible or widely understood.

Thus, it may not be a good indication of the public's response to more extensive use of general revenue financing.

Substantially increasing the general revenue share of Medicare financing may also be politically difficult when the federal government is facing large budget deficits. Any financing that is not closely linked to Medicare conceptually is likely to be vulnerable to criticism during periods of budgetary stringency. Unfortunately, all of the following proposals share this basic defect.

Earmarked Income Tax Surcharge

A 1 percent surcharge on individual income tax liabilities would raise about $5 billion in 1991, and a corporate income tax surcharge of 1 percent would raise about $1 billion. Assigning the revenue collected to the Medicare trust funds might serve to increase the political acceptability of such a surcharge. With continuing cutbacks in a variety of federal programs, however, there are many competing claims on additional general revenues.

Increased Alcohol and Tobacco Excise Taxes

Some portion of alcohol and tobacco excise taxes could be devoted to the Medicare trust funds. Consumption of these items affects health, and health status determines the usage of Medicare services. The relationship between heavy smoking and increased lung and heart disease is well established, as is the relationship between excessive use of alcohol and cirrhosis of the liver, certain cancers and highway injuries. Increasing excise taxes on alcohol and tobacco could be viewed as advance payment by those who smoke and drink for the higher medical costs that they, as a group, will incur, and because the administrative mechanism for collecting these taxes is already in place, there would be no additional administrative problems or costs.

Doubling federal excise taxes on alcohol (beer, wine, and distilled spirits) would raise about $6 billion in 1991, while doubling the $0.16 per pack tax on cigarettes would raise an additional $5 billion. The excise taxes on alcohol and tobacco have not kept up with inflation—they are based on units sold rather than value—so that substantial tax increases could be justified on that basis alone.

However, the portion of extra medical expenses that actually falls on the Medicare program is uncertain, as many of them will occur before people become eligible for Medicare. Indeed, to the extent that smoking and drinking lead to deaths before age 65, Medicare costs are reduced.

Another difficulty is that excise taxes are regressive; lower-income consumers pay a higher share of their incomes for these products than do higher-income consumers. Lastly, these taxes are not necessarily a stable source of revenue because smoking and drinking may decline as people become more concerned about their health. This decline would probably be encouraged by the higher costs the increased tax would impose.

Conclusion

If additional revenue to finance Medicare is needed, simply increasing the payroll tax ranks highest in terms of administrative simplicity and preservation of the insurance character of Medicare. Its regressive nature could be offset for lower-income workers by an increase in the earned income tax credit. The payroll tax is especially attractive if large amounts of money must be raised quickly.

Reallocating a portion of the projected OASDI trust fund surplus to Medicare would use up part of a fund that is being set aside to pay for the retirement benefits of the baby-boom generation. Reducing that fund could require lower benefits or higher payroll taxes in the years after 2020 and might reduce the confidence of the baby-boom generation in the Social Security system.

Some provisions, such as applying the Medicare payroll tax to state and local workers, make sense on their own merits, in addition to their contribution to Medicare financing. Other provisions are appealing only if changes are first made elsewhere in the tax system. Applying the Medicare payroll tax to all employee noncash benefits, taxing the insurance value of Medicare benefits and taxing Medigap premiums are probably only feasible administratively and politically if fringe benefits, including private health insurance, are first subjected to the individual income tax.

Proposals for financing Medicare that are not closely related to the program by either logic or history risk undermining the political support for Medicare. Proposals falling in this category include income tax surcharges and, perhaps, increased excise taxes on cigarettes and alcohol as well as elimination of the higher income tax standard deduction for the elderly.

Although all these financing options have their disadvantages, the support shown for the Medicare program over the years suggests a basic willingness to pay the costs of the benefits the public believes are necessary. The specific details of financing may in the end be less important than the perceived value of Medicare benefits, but careful thought on financing issues can prevent unnecessary erosion of public support.

NOTES

1. Unless otherwise noted, figures quoted are for alternative II-B of the Social Security Administration, Office of the Actuary, *1987 Annual Report of the Board of Trustees of the Federal Hospital Insurance Trust Fund.*

2. The general revenue transfer compensated the system for gratuitous military service wage credits as required under the 1983 Social Security Amendments.

3. The OASI trust fund repaid $1.8 billion of its $12.4 billion load to the HI trust fund in 1985. The remainder was repaid in 1986.

4. The term *general revenues* refers to all federal revenues other than those paid into trust funds.

5. The Tax Equity and Fiscal Responsibility Act (TEFRA) of 1982 required that the premium amount be calculated to produce premium income equal to 25 percent of program costs for 1984 and 1985. The Deficit Reduction Act of 1984 extended this requirement to 1987, after which the premium will increase in line with Old-Age, Survivors and Disability Insurance (OASDI) cost-of-living adjustments.

6. Because Medicare's major financing problems are projected to begin in the mid-1990s, it would be preferable to have longer-term estimates of the revenue impacts of the options discussed here. Unfortunately, estimates beyond 1991 are not currently available.

7. For further discussion of this option, see Munnell, 1985, pp. 52–56.

8. The extra "premium" could not be targeted with complete precision on Medicare beneficiaries because some elderly who would lose the deduction might not be covered by Medicare (for example, some former state and local workers).

9. Under the most progressive incidence assumptions in a recent study by Joseph Pechman (Pechman, 1985, p. 80), the estimated effective personal income tax rate in 1985 increased from 3.8 percent in the lowest tenth of the population to 13.5 percent in the highest tenth. The corporate income tax rate went from 1.6 percent to 3.6 percent. By contrast, the payroll tax rate went from 2.3 percent in the lowest tenth to 4.1 in the highest.

REFERENCES

Consolidated Omnibus Budget Reconciliation Act of 1985, Publ. L. No. 99–272, Sec. 13205 (100 Stat.) 313 (April 7, 1986).

Munnell, Alicia H. 1985. Paying for the Medicare Program. *New England Economic Review* January/February 46–66..

Munnell, A. H., and Lynn E. Blais. 1984. Do We Want Large Social Security Surpluses? *New England Economic Review* September/October 5–21.

Pechman, J. A. 1985. *Who Paid the Taxes, 1966–1985*. Washington: Brookings Institution.

Social Security Administration. 1986. Actuarial Note No. 127, Intermediate (Alternative II–B) Assumptions.

Social Security Administration. Office of the Actuary. 1987a. *1987 Annual Report of the Board of Trustees of the Federal Hospital Insurance Trust Fund.*

Social Security Administration. Office of the Actuary. 1987b. *1987 Annual Report of the Board of Trustees of the Supplementary Medical Insurance Trust Fund.*

U.S. Congressional Budget Office. 1986. *Reducing the Deficit: Spending and Revenue Options*. March.

U.S. Congressional Budget Office. 1987a. *Reducing the Deficit: Spending and Revenue Options*. January.

U.S. Congressional Budget Office. 1987b. *An Analysis of the President's Budgetary Proposals for Fiscal Year 1988*. February.

9

The Future of Medicare[1]

HARVARD MEDICARE PROJECT[2]

Since its enactment in 1965, Medicare has contributed a great deal to the health and welfare of the elderly and their families. Life expectancy at age 65 has increased two and one-half years. The elderly now see doctors at least as frequently as younger Americans. The middle generation no longer has to choose between providing for its children and financing health care for its parents.

Nevertheless, as the preceding chapters demonstrate, Medicare has a number of evident failings. The cost of physicians' services under Medicare continues to rise at an unacceptable rate. As of this writing, Medicare provides the elderly only the most minimal protection against the costs of catastrophic health care costs, though Congress may soon ameliorate this problem with new protections against catastrophic health care costs. Even these reforms, however, will leave the elderly vulnerable to the enormous, unpredictable and growing costs of long-term care. The elderly in 1987 paid a larger portion of their income for health care than they did before Medicare was enacted. The program has become so complicated that few elderly Americans understand how it works, what it entitles them to, or where to go to find out.

Based on the findings presented in the body of this volume, the Harvard Medicare Project sought solutions to these and other problems with the Medicare program. Our analysis is predicated on one premise and three goals.

The premise is that government must continue to play an important role in assuring that the elderly have adequate access to health care services and adequate protection against the costs of illness. Our goals are to promote cost control, fairness and simplicity in the Medicare program.

As in all other areas of social policy, it has become increasingly fashionable to address Medicare's problems with market-oriented solutions. We are neither opposed to private initiatives nor enamored of government. However, the special nature of older persons and their health problems argues for caution in relying primarily on private solutions to providing health care for them.

The Medicare program was enacted specifically because some elderly people were unable to obtain affordable private insurance. Today, this problem is even more severe. The costs of health care have soared and private insurers face sharply increased competition, thus making them less able to subsidize unprofitable enrollees.

Even when options are available, older persons may be unable to reap the benefits fully. As compared with younger consumers, the elderly are often less capable of making knowledgeable choices about health care purchases and less able to change vendors when dissatisfied. Partly because elderly persons are more likely to suffer physical and mental impairments (declining eyesight, hearing and memory), they have more trouble than younger Americans in comprehending the increasingly complex insurance arrangements now available. The elderly also usually lack the counsel of purchasing agents and benefits representatives who serve younger, employed populations. Although some retired Americans may be fully able to navigate our health care system, many others will not fair well in the rough and tumble of the health care marketplace.

Consequently, although we favor providing beneficiaries greater choice, we believe this can be best achieved by allowing elders more options within the existing Medicare program and by encouraging a cooperative approach between public and private sectors. Private health plans such as health maintenance organizations (HMOs) can play a more active role in the program. Government, however, must take an equally active role in making certain that the health care system provides the essential care that the elderly need. Recent reforms have demonstrated that Medicare can stimulate beneficial change in the way we pay for health services (through prospective hospital payments) and in the way health care is delivered (e.g., in hospices). Medicare should continue to have this role.

In discharging these responsibilities, the government should strive to achieve three goals. First, it is essential to contain Medicare's expenditures. Our concern is not only with the current federal deficit; rather, cost control is a valuable objective in its own right as long as it is achieved through changes that increase the efficiency of the program.

A second goal for the Medicare program is fairness to the elderly, to health care providers and to other groups (employers, insurance companies and family members) who are affected by the program. The elderly should receive affordable health care that is comparable in quality and amount to that enjoyed by the average American. Where cost considerations dictate limits on access to service or higher payments by beneficiaries, the burden should fall more heavily on the healthy and the wealthy.

Medicare should end payment policies that treat providers in capricious or unpredictable ways. The program should also honor its broader responsibility to society. It should pay enough to cover the reasonable costs of caring for its own beneficiaries, and it should promote payment systems that discourage discrimination against any group of patients.

A third goal of the Medicare program should be simplicity. Medicare is currently composed of several parts, each with its own procedural requirements and appeals processes. Beneficiaries must deal with five different types of cost sharing and seemingly arbitrary distinctions between covered and uncovered services. The Medicare program should be simplified so that both the elderly and their care givers can understand it.

With these principles in mind, the participants in the Harvard Medicare Project developed a set of recommendations designed to improve the performance of the Medicare program. These propose significant changes in the services the program covers, the cost sharing it requires of beneficiaries and the way it pays providers.

These are presented in two broad sets of reforms—those that affect beneficiaries and those that concern payment of health care providers.

Reforms Directly Affecting Beneficiaries

Three aspects of the Medicare program have direct and immediate effects on beneficiaries. The first is copayment responsibilities (coinsurance and deductibles), the amount beneficiaries must pay out-of-pocket at the time services are used. The second is the range of covered services, what Medicare will and will not help pay for. The third is the overall complexity of the system, which determines how easy or difficult it is for elderly people to use the Medicare program. In all three respects, Medicare can and should be improved.

Decrease Copayments, Increase Premiums

Present cost-sharing arrangements for Medicare patients are unfair and poorly conceived. Over the past 23 years, the proportion of Medicare costs paid through copayments has increased, whereas that paid through premiums (which are required only for Part B) has fallen. Monthly premiums have increased from $3.00 to roughly $17.90, but copayments and overall program costs have grown more than tenfold. Copayments disproportionately burden the poor and the sick, they have become excessive overall, and their unpredictability undermines the principles of insurance that Medicare was designed to promote (see Chapter 3).

To lessen or eliminate these drawbacks, we propose reducing or eliminating several of Medicare's deductible and coinsurance provisions and instituting a new, higher Medicare premium (which would incorporate the current Part B premium) paid by every enrollee to make up the lost revenues. We believe that the aggregate contribution of beneficiaries should be maintained at the current level of 25 percent of Medicare spending. We find premiums inherently preferable to coinsurance and deductibles for three reasons: Premiums are predictable, they do not penalize the sick and they can be related to income.

Specifically, we recommend that Medicare's hospital deductible, currently equivalent to the cost of a hospital day ($520), be cut in half; that the physician deductible (now $75) be eliminated; that the requirement that patients pay 25 percent of the cost of each hospital day after 60 days of hospitalization be eliminated; and that the physician coinsurance requirement be reduced from 20 percent to 10 percent. An additional annual payment of $150 to $200 for each beneficiary would offset both any revenues that were lost because of these changes as well as the costs of any additional health care.

The two forms of copayments that we would eliminate do little to control the use of health services; they only add to the amounts paid by elderly users of these services. Copayments for long hospital stays are no longer sensible now that Medicare's prospective payment system (PPS) creates incentives for early discharge. Physician deductibles are irrelevant to those beneficiaries (about half) whose chronic illnesses require that they see physicians frequently. These patients know that they will always spend far more than the deductible each year.

Even with the reduced coinsurance and deductible, copayments will accumulate into large bills for the very sick and the chronically ill elderly patients who use expensive services extensively (Waldo and Lazenby, 1984). This problem can be ameliorated by limiting each beneficiary's total annual liability for copayments to $1,000.

Adjust Cost Burden According to Ability to Pay

Increases in the premiums charged Medicare beneficiaries will disproportionately affect elderly persons with low incomes. To ease their burden, we propose, first, that uniform national standards be established for Medicaid's payment of Medicare premiums. Currently, because of varying state standards, only 25 percent of poor and near-poor elderly persons are covered by Medicaid, and states can refuse to purchase Medicare coverage (under Part B) even for those who are eligible to receive Medicaid. States should be required to pay the premiums for Medicare coverage for all elderly whose incomes are at or below 125 percent of the federal poverty level.

Second, we recommend assessing all taxpayers 65 and over a surtax equal to 5 percent of their income taxes. This reform would generate about $4 billion annually. Because only a little over 40 percent of the elderly pay income taxes at all, most of the added funds would be collected from those most able to pay. Among those affected, higher-income elderly would pay more than those with lower incomes. The additional revenues would be earmarked for the Medicare program and used to partially finance the premium to be paid by all beneficiaries. This would enable Medicare to set the premium at an amount that middle- and lower-income beneficiaries can afford to pay, one that is only slightly higher than the present Part B premium.

Public Supplementary Policy

More than half of all Medicare beneficiaries purchase private health insurance (Medigap) plans that eliminate or reduce liability for copayments. These plans are expensive, in part because of high administrative charges. Yet, many Medigap plans have limited value because they only duplicate existing Medicare coverage. Furthermore, because most private Medigap plans cover copayments, they eliminate any financial incentive beneficiaries have to limit their use of health care. Most of the resulting increase in use of services is paid for by the Medicare program rather than the private insurer, which means that Medicare inadvertently subsidizes the purchase of these plans.

We propose that a new Medicare-sponsored insurance policy be established that beneficiaries could purchase voluntarily. This policy should require nominal copayments of beneficiaries (e.g., a $50 hospital deductible and 5 percent coinsurance for physicians' services) and would be fully financed out of premiums paid by those who purchase the plan. In addition, we recommend that the federal government levy an excise tax on private Medigap plans so that their price will reflect the additional cost of the health care use they encourage.

Expanded Coverage of Long-Term Care and Chronic Illness

Even though about 25 percent of the health care costs for elderly persons are for long-term care services, Medicare now pays only a small part of the nursing home care and virtually none of the outpatient care of the chronically ill elderly that is provided by nonphysicians. For those who are eligible, Medicaid pays some of these costs. However, its coverage is incomplete, and eligibility requirements vary greatly from state to state. In many states, elders must impoverish themselves and their households before they become eligible for the Medicaid program.

As a society, we cannot in good conscience continue to deal with chronic illness in this manner. It robs the elderly of their dignity and of any real hope of economic and emotional security. Although we recognize that private insurers have begun to experiment with plans that cover some of the costs of nursing home care, there are three major reasons why the private market has failed, and will continue to fail, to offer reasonably priced insurance for long-term care.

First, few individuals are likely to purchase coverage until they reach their mid-70s, at a time when they must face the prospect that they may, in fact, need nursing home care (Johnson and Grant, 1985; Soldo and Manton, 1985). For most persons of that age, private insurance for nursing home care is too expensive. Premiums for a moderately comprehensive policy, covering nursing home care without requiring prior hospitalization and little home care can cost a 75-year-old more than $3,500 a year.[3] Second, because private companies fear that covered patients will overuse insured services, many of them will not offer coverage for a full range of noninstitutional care or they will price such coverage beyond the reach of all but a few wealthy persons (Lifson, 1984). Third, the marketing of insurance on an individual basis, which is necessary for most retirees, tends to make policies even more costly.

In many ways, the problem of long-term care that now faces elderly persons closely resembles the problem they had with physician and hospital services that led to the enactment of Medicare—the costs are high, the needs are pressing and the response of private insurers is insufficient.

To address the long-term care issue, we propose two major reforms in the Medicare program. First, Medicare should cover the cost of extended nursing home care (in addition to the limited, rehabilitative stays it currently covers), the single largest out-of-pocket health care expense for the elderly today. This coverage should be mandatory, and it should ultimately be financed in the same way as the rest of the Medicare program—that is, through a combination of Social Security taxes levied on the working population, premiums paid by elderly persons and general revenues.

Our proposal that Medicare cover nursing home care in this fashion raises a number of legitimate concerns. First, much of the cost of a nursing home represents living expenses (room and board), and many consider payment of such expenses by Medicare to be inappropriate. We propose that Medicare beneficiaries in nursing homes cover such nonmedical costs by making residential copayments equal to 80 percent of their Social Security benefits (Bishop, 1981).

Another concern is that covered nursing home services will be used inappropriately and excessively. The proposed residential copayment will partly discourage overuse, but we also suggest that Medicare beneficiaries be required to pay a deductible for extended nursing home care (beyond that currently covered by Medicare in full) equal to the cost of one month of care. Furthermore, we suggest that the Medicare program designate geriatric assessment teams of physicians, social workers and nurses in each community to act as gatekeepers. All admissions to nursing homes will require advance approval from those teams.

Our second major proposal is that Medicare provide more generous coverage of long-term care in outpatient settings, especially home health care and mental health services. Partly because of limitations on Medicare coverage, mentally ill older persons are now only half as likely to be treated as their younger counterparts (Shapiro et al., 1985). Furthermore, 10 to 30 percent of the elderly persons in nursing homes are there because they cannot find adequate outpatient services (Morris and Youket, 1981). To prevent the excessive use of these long-term care benefits, the community-based gatekeepers should also determine eligibility for these services.

Despite financial and administrative safeguards, an increase in coverage for nursing home care and chronic illnesses would be expensive. Additional expenditures could reach nearly $15 billion a year (in 1985 dollars) within 10 years after implementation (Table 9–1). We think that these costs are justified, but to accommodate concerns about the federal deficit, we suggest that these new benefits begin after current efforts to reduce the deficit have had time to take effect.

Improved Primary Care

Good primary care involves timely diagnosis and treatment. Eliminating the deductible on physician services, as suggested earlier, will remove an important barrier to such care. We propose further that Medicare cover an annual physical exam with no patient copayment. This visit should be limited to a set of specified, preventive screening tests such as cervical Papanicolaou smears, blood pressure checks, choles-

TABLE 9–1 Projected Societal Costs for Long-Term Care Under Present System and Proposed Medicare Coverage Beginning in 1990 (billions of 1985 dollars)

Type of Care	*1990*	*1995*	*2000*
Under Present System			
Nursing home care	$30.3	$34.5	$38.8
Outpatient chronic care[a]	5.3	5.9	6.6
Total cost	35.6	40.4	45.4
Under Proposed System			
Nursing home care[b]	30.3	45.8	50.4
Outpatient chronic care	7.3	8.2	9.4
Total cost	37.6	54.0	59.8
Difference between present and proposed coverages	2.0	13.6	14.4

[a]Includes home health care and outpatient mental health care.

[b]In 1990, nursing home utilization is assumed to be limited by available supply of beds. By 1995, the supply is assumed to rise to meet the following changes in utilization: (1) 20 percent of those who would otherwise be in nursing homes are assumed to remain in the community owing to enhanced home care; (2) all elders who require personal care (eating, toileting, dressing) and who are unmarried or living alone are placed in homes; (3) half of the elders with impaired mobility who are living alone are placed in homes.

Sources: Survey-based data on impairment in elderly populations (Weissert, 1985); nursing home use (Rice and Feldman, 1983; Weissert, 1985); home health care use (Hicks et al., 1981; Manton and Liu, 1984); and the use of mental health services (Shapiro et al., 1985; Sharfstein, et al., 1984). Data on senior utilization drawn from elderly population (Morris and Youket, 1981); nursing home use (Morris and Youket, 1981; Weissert, 1985); home health care use (Rice and Feldman, 1983; Manton and Liu, 1984); and mental health utilization (Hicks et al., 1981; Lane, 1986).

terol determinations, rectal exams and stool assessments for occult blood. For persons who are unable to visit a physician's office, Medicare should pay home health agencies to conduct similar examinations.

Administrative Simplification

Many of the proposals we have discussed would, if enacted, help to simplify the Medicare program for beneficiaries. Their responsibilities for copayments would become simpler and easier to understand. The arbitrary coverage distinctions between acute and chronic care and between physical and mental illness would be eliminated.

To simplify the program further we propose that Medicare's Parts A and B (which cover hospital and nonhospital services, respectively) should be combined into a single unified program that would enable Medicare to offer older persons a uniform structure of benefits and cost-sharing requirements.

In addition to a simplified program structure, elderly persons need advocates and easy sources of information about the Medicare program. As efforts mount to control program costs through prospective payment, Medicare beneficiaries may be denied care by providers (see Chapter 5). As the number of new insurance plans (e.g., HMOs) available to Medicare beneficiaries grows, elderly persons also face a confusing array of options in coverage and copayments. We propose that Medicare pay for the support of a Medicare ombudsman's office within each Area Agency on Aging. The ombudsman's job would be to provide beneficiaries with information on their rights and options under Medicare, to assist beneficiaries with paperwork, to transmit complaints and to monitor and review beneficiaries' access to care.

Financial Impact of Proposed Reforms

If all the reforms proposed here were adopted, they would change the health care costs faced by beneficiaries in two ways. Expanded coverage and reduced copayments would decrease the total costs that the elderly now pay out-of-pocket for all health care, including nursing home care (Table 9–2). By changing the methods of

TABLE 9–2 Projected Financial Impact of Reforms on Beneficiaries (1985 dollars)

		2000	
	1990	*Excluding Long Term Care*	*Including Long Term Care*
Beneficiary share of new Medicare expenditures—added costs	$1.1 billion	$280 million	$11.3 billion
Beneficiary savings from coverage of previously uncovered costs	2.3 billion	3.5 billion	11.2 billion
Beneficiary savings owing to broader Medicaid coverage	—	2.3 billion	3.9 billion
Net financial impact on beneficiaries—savings	1.2 billion	5.5 billion	3.8 billion

Based on calculations described in appendix to this chapter.

financing elders' contributions to program expenditures, the proposals also redistribute the Medicare cost burden from poor to wealthier beneficiaries.

Considered together, the proposed reforms will considerably decrease the cost burden on elders with incomes in the lowest quartile. By reducing copayments and by ensuring that Medicaid purchases their Medicare premiums, the health care costs of this group will decline from between 25 and 30 percent of income to 10 to 15 percent. Elders with incomes in the second lowest quartile will also benefit. They will pay substantially lower copayments, only slightly increased premiums, and—because their incomes are low enough that they generally do not have taxable incomes—they will pay for little of the earmarked income tax revenues for the program.

Elders with above average incomes will pay more under the proposed changes. Income taxes earmarked for the Medicare program will require an additional 2 to 3 percent of their income. Even with these changes, however, beneficiaries with incomes in these ranges will pay between 7 to 10 percent of income for health care expenses, including coverage of long-term care. This seems a reasonable share of costs and is still less than that borne by elders with lower incomes.

Reforms in Payment of Providers

Physicians

Current methods for paying physicians under Medicare have a number of drawbacks that contribute to escalating costs and the unfair treatment of beneficiaries and physicians alike.

From the beginning, Medicare has reimbursed physicians according to the customary, prevailing and reasonable (CPR) method. For several reasons, this system has contributed to escalating costs (see Chapter 6). First, because it pays physicians on a fee-for service basis, it creates a built-in incentive for physicians to provide more services. Because payment is based partly on what physicians customarily charge, the method has perpetuated the relatively high fees specialists and surgeons charge, thus encouraging such physicians to provide more high-technology services.

The Medicare payment system is also unfair to patients in that it allows physicians to accept or reject assignment (i.e., to decide whether to accept the fee set by Medicare as full compensation) on a case-by-case basis. Physicians who refuse assignment must bill the patient directly to get paid, but they may then charge more than the fee set by Medicare. Ten percent of beneficiaries' out-of-pocket spending for physicians' services in 1983 were payments for unassigned charges. Such expenditures add to the confusion of elderly patients, they impair access to care and they vary arbitrarily from physician to physician and region to region.

The current system for paying physicians also tends to treat certain groups of physicians unfairly. Even when specialists and surgeons provide services that are similar to those given by primary care practitioners, they receive more compensation. In 1982, for example, specialists were paid 20 to 53 percent more for a brief office visit than were primary care physicians. Physicians in urban areas are generally paid considerably more than physicians in rural areas.

To ameliorate these problems of cost and fairness, we recommend that Medicare pursue four major avenues of reform. First, the program should continue to encourage enrollment in prepaid health care organizations (discussed later). However, we recommend caution in implementing systems that reimburse individual physicians for ambulatory services alone on a prepaid basis under managed-care arrangements. Without the financial resources and management expertise that are available to large organizations, individual physicians might not be effective in containing costs while preserving the quality of care.

As long as enrollment in prepaid health care organizations remains voluntary for Medicare beneficiaries, many—perhaps most—will continue to be cared for by physicians on a fee-for-service basis. Some way must be found, therefore, to improve on the CPR methodology in determining fee-for-service payments. Thus, as a second major reform, we recommend that Medicare pay physicians according to a relative value scale that is adjusted by a dollar-value multiplier. A properly designed relative value scale could help control costs by making physician payments fiscally neutral. It would reduce fees for certain services that are now expensive and overvalued under the CPR system (such as certain speciality services). Such a system would also eliminate unjustifiable differences in fees charged to beneficiaries and paid to physicians in different geographic regions. To help ensure that the process of establishing the system is open and deliberative and that the concerned parties are represented, we recommend that an expert national commission with physician representation be formed to devise the fee schedule.

To simplify the work of developing a relative value fee schedule and to help control overall costs, the first task of the national commission should be to reduce the number of separate items for which physicians can bill Medicare. Currently, physicians may bill Medicare separately for any item included in the American Medical Association's listing of services and procedures, the "Current Procedures Terminology" (CPT). There are now 7,500 items in the CPT, almost four times as many as in 1966. The complexity of the code permits physicians considerable latitude in billing for similiar services, and there is an obvious temptation to choose the billing code for which the fee is the highest. Moreover, it is relatively easy to break down a single service into several billable services. The national commission should reduce the number of items in the CPT to fewer than 1000.

Because any fee-for-service system encourages physicians to deliver more services, the implementation of a relative value scale would not guarantee overall cost savings to the program. Thus, to ensure that such savings occur, we recommend, as part of a third major reform, that the federal government establish an annual budget target for total expenditures for physicians' services under Medicare. If payments exceeded that target in any year, the federal government could reduce the dollar-value multipliers for the following year by an amount that would be sufficient to recover the excess.

As a fourth major change in physician reimbursement, we recommend that Medicare require physicians to accept assignment—that is, accept Medicare's fee as payment in full (less any coinsurance and deductibles)—for all beneficiaries. Neither patients nor physicians should be eligible to receive Medicare payment for services rendered by physicians who refuse assignment. Failing to adopt mandatory assignment would undermine the effectiveness of a fee schedule based on relative values because physicians who were dissatisfied with the fees paid by Medicare could charge patients whatever the fee schedule denied them. Unfortunately, immediate introduction of mandatory assignment could adversely affect access to care under Medicare. Physicians in certain areas might simply refuse to treat Medicare beneficiaries. Thus, this change in payment policy should be implemented gradually over 5 to 10 years, and it should start with mandatory assignment for all physicians' services to hospitalized patients. Assignment should eventually be made mandatory for all outpatient charges as well.

Hospitals

Medicare's current prospective payment system (PPS), a system of regulated prices based on diagnosis-related groups (DRGs), is almost certainly an improvement over the cost-based approach to reimbursement that preceded it. Though the implementation of the PPS does not deserve all the credit for recent declines in the rate of increase in hospital costs, it has contributed to growing cost consciousness among the nation's hospitals.

Nevertheless, the current PPS has a number of flaws. First, it controls the amount paid for a hospital admission but not the number of patients a hospital can admit. Because hospitals can thus boost revenues by increasing admissions of Medicare beneficiaries, the PPS may not be effective in controlling costs in the long run.

Second, Medicare's current prospective payment system may promote discrimination against certain groups of patients. Because that system controls only Medicare prices, it may make elderly patients less desirable than privately insured persons, leading to a tendency to discharge Medicare beneficiaries sicker and quicker than other individuals. The PPS will encourage hospitals to favor admission of Medicare patients who are in more profitable diagnostic groups and who are less severely ill. Uninsured patients also suffer under this system as it is increasingly difficult to cross-subsidize their care from hidden surpluses built into Medicare and other fees.

We think that better prospective payment systems can be designed. We propose one here that should be considered if flaws in the current PPS create pressure for major reform. We recommend a system of prospectively set budget targets for hospitals that includes safeguards against discrimination against Medicare and uninsured patients. The fundamentals of this approach are discussed below.

Each year, the federal government should set a target budget for hospital payments for each state. The states should then be empowered to devise ways to keep Medicare hospital costs within that target or they should be required to make up the difference from their own resources. To achieve this goal, the states should have wide discretion in determining how hospitals within their boundaries will be paid for providing services to Medicare beneficiaries.

In designing payment systems, however, the states should meet certain federal requirements. All payers within their jurisdiction should use the same method for paying for hospital care and rates for different payers should reflect the costs of treating such patients—not the market power or negotiating skill of the payers. State authorities should negotiate with each hospital a limit on the institution's total revenues from all sources for the next year. If those budget targets are exceeded, then the hospitals involved should be paid at a reduced rate for the rest of the year. The states should also be required to establish systems to cover the costs of caring for uninsured patients. Medicare should contribute its fair share to such uncompensated care schemes. Finally, the federal government should oversee state implementation of the new payment system to assure that no state system discriminates against any class of payers or any racial or ethnic group.

Experience in this country and abroad (e.g., Massachusetts and Canada) has demonstrated that such a system is workable and that it can constrain the rise in overall hospital costs.[4] Because this system limits hospital budgets instead of Medicare prices, it promises to be a better method than the current PPS for reducing the rate of growth in hospital costs over the long term. By limiting increases in hospital expenditures for both private and public patients, the system would use Medicare's leverage in the health care system to limit the growth in all health care costs, not just Medicare expenditures. In addition, because it would create an all-payers system, the plan would ensure that Medicare patients were treated as fairly as other consumers of hospital services. Finally, the proposed plan would provide federal leadership in designing solutions to the growing problem of providing uninsured patients with access to hospital care.

Prepaid Health Care

Sixty years of experience and research have documented the ability of HMOs to deliver high-quality care at costs that are lower than those in the fee-for-service sector. Allowing Medicare beneficiaries to choose among prepaid plans expands their options, thereby encouraging innovation and enabling beneficiaries to find plans that cover services that best meet their needs.

Nevertheless, as most of our experience with HMOs involves working populations rather than retirees, some caution is indicated in applying that experience to the Medicare population. The very high costs of caring for some elderly patients may encourage prepaid health care organizations to selectively enroll healthy Medicare patients, channelling more costly patients into the fee-for-service system. If HMOs are paid the average cost of treating a Medicare patient in the traditional system, but they enroll only patients who are healthier than average, overall Medicare expenses may increase and care of the healthiest elders may be inappropriately subsidized.

The track record of HMOs is, however, long and strong enough to justify encouraging increased enrollment of Medicare beneficiaries in them. The Medicare amendments of 1982 took a major step in this direction by reimbursing HMOs at 95 percent of the average age/sex adjusted Medicare payments (AAPCC) in the communities where they are located. To encourage additional enrollment Medicare should allow HMOs to recruit up to 75 percent of their members from the Medicare population (the limit is now 50 percent). This would permit specialization in the health needs of the elderly without taking that group of patients completely out of the mainstream of care.

If the Medicare program and its beneficiaries are to benefit fully from the option to choose among HMOs, it is essential to promote informed decisions and to discourage selective enrollment of healthy older persons. Medicare should provide beneficiaries with easily understandable information about the benefit packages and costs of all participating HMOs. We recommend that the Health Care Financing Administration (HCFA) establish standardized estimates of the expected monetary value of Medicare benefits offered by HMOs. All marketing material and written advertisements issued by participating HMOs should include the estimated value of a range of health services—both those that are offered by a particular plan and those that are not. To make certain that the elderly have easy access to prepaid organizations, we also recommend that the Social Security Administration annually distribute the above information on HMOs to all beneficiaries. Direct mailing of information—coupled with the current requirement that HMOs have open-enrollment periods—will limit the ability of plans to market selectively.

Improved methods for setting AAPCC rates, upon which Medicare bases payment of prepaid plans, should be developed at the earliest possible date. Incorporating measures such as beneficiaries' past health care expenses and their current health status would help adjust AAPCC rates to reflect the actual cost of treating Medicare beneficiaries in a given community. More accurate payment rates would counteract incentives for HMOs to avoid enrolling the sickest elders and to stint on costly services such as those involved in the treatment of chronic illness.

Because adequate adjustment of the AAPCC is not likely to be feasible in the near future, Congress should act immediately to provide for better balanced risk sharing between individual HMOs and the Medicare program. The program should provide HMOs with reinsurance against large losses on Medicare contracts as well as share more directly in the cost savings if a plan enrolls unusually healthy elders. In either case, sharing of costs and savings should be based on audits of actual expenditures that HMOs incur providing care for Medicare beneficiaries.

Medicare should also monitor the performance of HMOs. Currently, professional review organizations (PROs) oversee the quality of hospital care to counteract similar incentives under the PPS. The PROs or some other competent outside agency should do the same for HMOs.

Finally, because many elders need a combination of health care and social services, Medicare should encourage the development of social/health maintenance organizations (S/HMOs) that draw on both Medicare coverage and funding from such programs as Medicaid, Title III of the Older Americans Act and Title XX of the Social Security Act. As with most experiments, the initial costs may be high. We suggest that Congress consider subsidizing the capitalization of such plans, in much the same way that HMOs were federally subsidized in the mid-1970s.

Implementing the Medicare Reform Proposal

We have tried to develop an integrated set of proposals, one in which the reforms affecting beneficiaries are compatible with those affecting providers and those dealing with the structure of the program. These reforms represent a blueprint for a Medicare program which would, through the year 2000, serve the needs of beneficiaries while making the Medicare program a socially responsible part of the health care system.

We do not, however, think it either feasible or wise to implement all these reforms simultaneously. A number of our proposals cannot be enacted immediately. Some require the development of new methods of paying providers or assessing the health of beneficiaries; such innovations, although feasible, will take time. Other reforms will require substantial added federal spending. Though we believe that these reforms can be fairly and adequately financed, it appears impractical to introduce them at a time when federal spending is being cut to eliminate a huge deficit. We therefore recommend full-scale implementation of these more costly programs only after current initiatives to balance the federal budget have had some success.

A number of other proposals, however, could and should be enacted more quickly. These require no major technical breakthroughs, will not add significantly to the costs of the Medicare program and need not be coordinated with other proposals that must be phased in more slowly. We believe that they will significantly improve the lot of Medicare's beneficiaries and promote a better-functioning program.

Because the interactions among the various reforms are complex and because all predictions about the future are somewhat uncertain, determining the appropriate time to initiate a particular reform is difficult. Nonetheless, we think it helpful to convey our sense of when our proposed changes could reasonably be integrated into Medicare. To do so, we have divided the discussion of implementation into three phases: reforms that can be implemented over the next five years, reforms that can be implemented between 5 and 10 years from now, and reforms requiring 10 to 15 years for implementation. These three steps are summarized in Table 9–3.

Phase 1: 1 to 5 Years

Many of our proposals can be implemented by making simple changes in administration of the program. Because these reforms do not rely on complicated changes in the structure of the health care system, they can be implemented fairly rapidly. A number of the proposals earmarked for this stage are designed to redistribute beneficiaries' share of costs from copayments to premiums, thus making these costs more predictable and better matched to elders' incomes. By reducing the types of copayments and making a small number of changes in program structure, we hope to simplify the program for beneficiaries. We also propose adopting a set of procedural reforms in this stage that will promote enrollment in HMOs and provide some assurance that such enrollment benefits both elders and the Medicare program.

As noted in the discussion of reforms, a number of other proposals require refinements of current methods of health assessment or health care delivery. We therefore also propose that a series of demonstration projects take place in this initial 5-year period. These include experimenting with the organization and payment of interdisciplinary geriatric assessment teams, with incentive payment arrangements for case managers of long-term-care benefits, with methods of adjusting the AAPCC for individual differences in health status and with procedures for standardizing marketing of competing HMOs.

Phase 2: 5 to 10 Years

During the second phase, we propose completing cost-sharing reforms by instituting limits on future increases in copayments and creating uniform national standards for elders' eligibility under Medicaid. Mandatory assignment of physicians' charges—initiated for inpatient fees in Phase 1—should be extended to large outpatient bills in Phase 2. In addition, where demonstrations were initiated in Phase 1, their findings can be fully integrated into the Medicare program at this stage.

TABLE 9–3 Schedule for Implementing Reforms

Category of Reform	Phase 1 (1 to 5 years)	Phase 2 (5 to 10 years)	Phase 3 (10 to 15 years)
Cost sharing	Reductions in copayments Optional supplementary coverage Ceiling on copayment liability	Limits to copayment increases Uniform national eligibility under Medicaid at 125% of poverty line	
Service coverage	Physician diagnostic visit Diagnostic visit by home health agencies Long-term care case-management demonstration projects	Begin phase-in of coverage of long-term-care services Interdisciplinary geriatric assessments	Complete coverage of long-term-care services
Simplification	Combine Parts A and B Institute Medicare ombudsman		
Physician payment	Mandatory assignment of inpatient charges	Physician choice of outpatient assignment for all patients or none Adopt relative value scale for physician payments Demonstration projects in physician all-payers systems	Mandatory assignment of all charges
Hospital payment		Medicare accepts responsibility for paying for share of uncompensated care Begin phase-in of state-based all-payers systems Begin phase-in of hospital-based budgets for Medicare	Complete phase-in of all-payers systems Complete phase-in of hospital budgets
Prepaid health plans	More flexible restrictions on enrollment and retained earnings Standardized marketing demonstration projects Active oversight by PROs Better balanced rise sharing	Incorporate adjustments for health status into AAPCC Standardized marketing regulations	
Financing of program	Earmarked income tax revenues from beneficiaries	Increase in earned income tax credit (as payroll tax increases to pay for long-term-care coverage)	

The majority of the reforms introduced in this phase, however, are associated with three major initiatives: coverage of long-term care, payment of physicians under a relative value scale, adoption of hospital reimbursement reforms based on all-payers systems and budget targets for each institution. Each of these proposals is initiated in Phase 2 for somewhat different reasons. Long-term-care coverage is delayed because it will require additional governmental spending (and thus is incompatible with current efforts to reduce federal spending). It also relies on a gatekeeping role for geriatric assessment teams, which will be refined in the first stage of implementation. As an adjunct to long-term-care coverage, evaluation of beneficiaries by interdisciplinary geriatric assessment teams will also be covered in this period. The relative value system for physician payment is currently undergoing further study and refinement; results of this research will not be available for several years. Finally, although we foresee a clear need for some form of prospective budgeting for hospital payment, we anticipate that the shortcomings of the current PPS system will not become generally evident until there is an end to the ongoing secular decline of hospital admissions. At that point, we expect that the limitations of DRGs will lead to political support for more comprehensive reimbursement reforms.

Phase 3: 10 to 15 Years

A number of the large-scale reforms, including all-inclusive mandatory assignment of the physicians' charges, coverage of long-term care and prospective budgeting for hospital care, will require a number of years to implement fully. This phased implementation is completed in the third stage of our proposal. Such delays are more realistic than, and preferable to, more rapid introduction of reforms. We believe that at the end of this 15-year period, the Medicare program will be financially stable, structured to meet the major needs of beneficiaries and equipped to adapt to changes in the health care system in the year 2000 and beyond.

We have tried to provide such a coherent vision in this chapter. It is motivated most fundamentally by our assessment of the needs and concerns of America's elders. Whatever Medicare's other attributes, it should first and foremost be a program that truly serves its beneficiaries. To this end, we have recommended changes in service coverage that reflect the health care needs of elder patients. We suggest simplifying the program, so that it can be fully comprehended and effectively used by its beneficiaries. We further propose administrative changes, such as the creation of a Medicare ombudsman's office, that would aid elders who are in need of information or who believe that they have been unfairly treated by health care providers or fiscal intermediaries.

In designing this plan, we rejected some reforms that would clearly have improved elders' welfare. In some cases, we did this because we anticipated that the reforms would diffuse Medicare's orientation as a health care program and thus potentially undermine its political support. In other cases, we judged that the costs of reforms would be excessive, or that the risk of uncontrollable spending on these proposals was simply too high. Our choices have been disciplined by the self-imposed requirement that the savings generated by reforms in provider payment should cover the costs of additional acute care benefits.

Medicare and Future Reform

In many ways, the Medicare program has aged gracefully over the past twenty-three years. It continues to serve well many of its beneficiaries. It has maintained widespread public support among older and younger Americans. But time has left its marks. Changing conditions among the elderly and within the health care system have exacerbated flaws inherent in the program since its inception. If not addressed, these will diminish Medicare's capacity to address the important health care needs of its beneficiaries.

As these failings have become more apparent, calls for reform have increased. Congress is becoming more receptive, and a number of changes in Medicare are likely to be enacted over the next several years. Because the American political process favors incremental over comprehensive reform, these changes will probably take the form of a series of individually modest amendments to the program. In addition to catastrophic coverage, these measures are likely to include continued adjustment of the prospective payment system for hospitals, some reforms in physician payment, and attempts to better regulate the provision of prepaid services to Medicare patients.

Policymakers must not lose sight of the overall directions in which the Medicare program is evolving as these reforms are enacted. Piecemeal changes can be counterproductive if they work at cross-purposes or obscure more fundamental underlying problems with the program. A broader vision of the Medicare program is necessary if this reform process is to produce a more balanced and effective program.

Accurately predicting the costs of all our suggested reforms in the Medicare program—some of which would not be implemented for a number of years—is a hazardous enterprise. We have, however, made some preliminary estimates using methods described in the appendix to this chapter. Excluding additional long-term-care benefits, we estimate the financial impact of our proposals on Medicare expenditures in the year 2000 could range from a net savings of several billion dollars to a net loss of approximately $3 billion (in 1985 dollars), depending on the assumptions used (Harvard Medicare Project, 1986). As discussed earlier in this chapter (Table 9–1), coverage for chronic and nursing home care would increase Medicare's spending by roughly $50 billion annually, though $35 billion of this simply substitutes for costs that would have been paid by Medicaid or by elderly persons and their families.

It is imperative to consider these costs in assessing the merits of this package of proposals. Yet, it is just as essential to consider other factors that have received less attention in the current fiscal and political climate. Given the current drift of Medicare policy, what kind of protection against the financial costs of illness will elderly Americans have in the year 2000? What kind of access will they have to services? How will we care for the growing numbers of elderly persons who can no longer live alone?

These questions deserve consideration now if only because current changes in policy should be informed by long-range considerations. In 1965, the political process produced a Medicare program that, for all its current failings, represented a triumph of humane public policy. It is now time to correct those failings so that the program can meet the challenges of the next 20 years.

NOTES

1. Portions of this chapter were previously published in the *New England Journal of Medicine* ("The Future of Medicare," by David Blumenthal, Mark Schlesinger, and Pamela Brown Drumheller, 314 (11):722–28, March 13, 1986) and are used here with the permission of the *New England Journal of Medicine*.

2. Funds for the Harvard Medicare Project were supplied by the Milbank Memorial Fund to the Division of Health Policy Research and Education at Harvard University. However, the opinions expressed herein are those of the participants of the Harvard Medicare Project only and should not be taken to represent the views of the Fund or of Harvard University.

3. In 1984, the average daily cost of skilled-nursing home care in Massachusetts was $75 (U.S. Congress, House Select Committee on Aging, 1985). For a 75-year-old, an Aetna nursing home policy (20-day deductible, no prior hospitalization required; home care covered only if after a 120 day stay in a nursing home) that would cover these charges would, in 1986, require premiums of $3,568 annually.

4. In 1983, the first year of Massachusetts's all-payer hospital reimbursement system (Chapter 372), both hospital costs and revenues increased significantly less in Massachusetts than in the rest of the country (and significantly less than during prior years in Massachusetts). Hospital patient services' revenues and costs increased by 8.1 percent and 6.7 percent in 1983, respectively, compared with national increases of approximately 13 percent for both revenues and costs. In 1984, hospital revenue and cost increases were 7.1 percent and 6.2 percent, respectively (Commonwealth of Massachusetts, 1986).

APPENDIX 9–A

Estimated Costs and Savings from Proposed Reforms

This appendix provides estimates of the fiscal impact of the proposed reforms and a brief description of the way in which these were calculated. Because we recommend phasing in a number of new programs, the aggregate cost of the reform package varies over time. We, therefore, present estimates for both 1990, after the initial phase of reform is completed, and 2000, by which time all the proposed changes could be integrated into the Medicare program.

In any projection of future costs, there is a good deal of uncertainty. Because a number of our proposed reforms involve new methods of payment, administrative procedures or coverage of previously uncovered services, accurate predictions are even more difficult. Thus, although we present specific estimates for each reform, it should be recognized that each is imprecise—on the order of plus or minus 25 percent for the average prediction. As a result, although we estimate that by the year 2000 the proposed savings of reforms of Medicare's coverage of acute care services will roughly offset the added costs of other reforms (Table 9–A1), it is possible in the worst case that net costs would increase by up to $5 billion. Conversely, in the best case, net program costs might fall by about $3 billion. (To avoid the uncertainties of predicting future rates of inflation all cost estimates in this appendix are presented in 1985 dollars.)

TABLE 9–A1 Projected Impact of Reforms on Medicare Program Expenditures[a] (in 1985 dollars)

		2000	
	1990	*Excluding Long-Term Care*	*Including Long-Term Care*
Expenditures for total program	$ 4.9 billion	$ 1.2 billion	$49.3 billion
Portion financed through			
General federal revenues[b]	1.1 billion	280 million	11.3 billion
Beneficiary contributions	1.1 billion	280 million	11.3 billion
State share of Medicaid Buy-in	100 million	25 million	1.0 billion
Payroll tax	2.6 billion	615 million	25.7 billion

[a]Excludes imposition of unified Medicaid coverage.

[b]These expenditures include the general revenues financing of the Medicare program and the federal portion of Medicaid costs.

Calculating Costs/Savings from Proposed Reforms

Baseline Projections

As a result of the overall aging of the American population, even in the absence of inflation, Medicare costs will continue to increase through the year 2000. Past studies predict that, if current patterns of utilization continue, hospital costs among the elderly would increase 35 to 40 percent between 1985 and 2000; physician costs would rise by about 30 percent and nursing home expenditures would grow 50 to 60 percent (Russell, 1981; Rice and Feldman, 1983). Consequently, with no changes in coverage, we would predict that Medicare spending on hospital care would rise to $59 billion annually by 1990 and to $70 billion by the year 2000 simply as the result of changing demographics. Spending on physician care would increase to $18 billion in 1990 and to $21 billion 10 years later (Table 9–A2).

Increased Spending from Cost-Sharing Reforms

By redistributing costs from copayments to premiums, our reforms will increase utilization and costs. The magnitude of this increase, however, is less than might have been expected. Research on Medicare beneficiaries who are exempt from copayments (either because they have purchased Medigap plans or are enrolled in Medicaid) indicates that their utilization is 30 to 50 percent higher (depending on type of service and health status) than comparable beneficiaries who do face copayments (Long et al., 1982).

Because our proposed reforms eliminate between two-thirds and three-quarters of copayment liability, one would predict—assuming that the impact of copayments is proportional to their size—that they would increase utilization and costs by 15 to 25 percent.

TABLE 9–A2 Breakdown of Added Costs or Cost Savings of Proposed Reforms in 1990 and 2000 (in 1985 dollars)

	Impact on Medicare Budget	
Type of Reform	*1990*	*2000*
Payments by Beneficiaries		
(1) Reduced copayment	$3.1 billion	$5.2 billion
(2) Capped beneficiary liability @ $1,000	1.4 billion	2.0 billion
Coverage of Services		
(1) Primary care improvement	500 million	3.4 billion
(2) Long-term care	NA[a]	47.8 billion
Program Simplification		
Uniform Medicaid eligibility (125% of poverty line)	NA[a]	—
Hospital Payment		
(1) Hospital budget caps	NA[a]	(5.7 billion)[b]
(2) Uncompensated care	NA[a]	4.3 billion
Physician Payment		
(1) Prospective pricing	NA[a]	(5.5 billion)[b]
(2) Mandatory assignment of Medicare charges	1.1 billion	1.5 billion
Alternative Payment Systems		
More representative HMO enrollment	(800 million)[b]	(4.0 billion)[b]

[a]NA: Not applicable, reform not yet initiated.

[b]Figures in parentheses indicate cost savings.

This holds true, however, only for beneficiaries who would otherwise have paid these copayments. Surveys indicate that only about one third of all beneficiaries fall into this category: The rest are fully or partially exempted from copayments as a result of Medigap or Medicaid coverage (Cafferata, 1984). The net impact of our reforms is thus much smaller, on the order of a 4-to-5-percent increase in physician utilization and a 6-to-8-percent increase in hospital costs.

Costs of Primary-Care-Improvement Package

For the most part the annual physician visit for preventive care would be used only by elders who did not otherwise see a doctor: 6 million elders in any given year, or 20 percent (U.S. Department of Health and Human Services, 1985). Some elders, though, might substitute this visit for a regular physical exam. Because beneficiaries with chronic illness have little financial incentive to do so, we anticipate that the maximum use of this coverage would reach about 15 million visits (all beneficiaries who do not need to see a physician for care of chronic illness). Most likely, coverage would involve some middle level of use. At $40 a visit for a limited examination, costs of coverage might run $400 million to $500 million each year.

If diagnostic visits by home health care agencies are limited to beneficiaries who have not seen a physician in 2 years, statistics indicate that 10 percent of the elderly population, about 3 million elders, would be eligible (U.S. Department of Health and Human Services, 1985). By further limiting services to those who are homebound, the eligible population would be made considerably smaller, though it is not clear by how much. At a maximum, assuming each visit cost $40, added coverage would cost on the order of $150 million annually.

There is, however, a clear substitution between these two services. The more elders who take advantage of the free physician visit, the fewer would be eligible for home diagnostic service. Thus, we anticipate that the combined annual costs of the two services will be about $500 million to $550 million.

The costs of the geriatric assessment team will depend on the number of seriously impaired elders who seek coverage under Medicate's long-term-care provisions and are referred for assessment. We expect this to amount to roughly 5 million in 1990, growing to 6 million by 2000 (Weissert, 1985). A limited number of demonstration projects suggest that assessment costs could run $250 to $500 a case. Assuming conservatively that the higher estimate is accurate, total costs of coverage would be between $2.5 billion and $3.0 billion annually.

Costs of Long-Term Care Coverage

Because there are no studies that can be used to reliably estimate the impact of price on demand for these services, predictions of their costs are based on estimates of need in the elderly population and the experience of a small number of demonstration projects such as the Triage program (Hicks et al., 1981). (Because use of these services requires prior authorization, need-based estimates are more reasonable upper bounds for long-term-care use than they would be for either hospital or physician care.)

As noted in Table 9–1, estimates of nursing home use are based on the following assumptions: (1) all elders needing assistance with personal care (eating, bathing, dressing or toileting) who are living alone or are unmarried go into a nursing home, (2) all the elders who have mobility limitations and who live alone go into nursing homes, and (3) 20 percent of those now in nursing homes are able to live in the community owing to improved home care. The assumptions represent a doubling in the rate of institutionalization of elders with personal-care needs and a sixfold increase in the institutionalization rate of elders with impaired mobility (Weissert, 1985). Under these assumptions, using existing projections of the number of elders with various levels of impairment but adjusting for future demographic changes, overall costs for nursing home care would be about $40 billion in 1990, $50 billion by the year 2000.

The experience of the Triage program suggests that relaxing the current limited acute care restrictions on home care could lead to between a doubling and tripling of use (Hicks et al., 1981). Because this program did not use copayments, as proposed here, we anticipate that use will likely double under our proposal, leading to costs of between $5.8 and $7.5 billion each year.

Use of mental health care services is most difficult to predict. Experience with coverage of younger populations, including the Rand Health Insurance Experiment, suggests that greater coverage (with moderate copayments), as proposed here, would lead to a doubling in use of services (Manning et al., 1986). Because this corresponds roughly to assessments of unmet mental health care needs in the elderly population, we use it as a crude prediction of future costs, amounting to between $700 million and $1 billion yearly. (The literature suggests that this will create a corresponding, though somewhat smaller, decrease in the use of general health care [Sharfstein et al., 1984]. To keep our estimates conservative, we have not included this offset in these calculations.)

Savings from Standardized Marketing of Prepaid Plans

The magnitude of the savings from these reforms depends both on the number of Medicare beneficiaries enrolled in HMOs and the potential for selective enrollment that now exists. Although some observers expect very rapid expansion of prepayment under Medicare, we have adopted a more conservative prediction: By 1990, 15 percent of all beneficiaries will be enrolled in HMOs, by the year 2000, 30 percent.

Recently published studies suggest that if prepaid plans successfully screen potential enrollees on the basis of prior health care utilization, they will enroll a population with costs 3 to 6 percent below average (Eggars and Prihoda, 1982). Other studies suggest that a small number of sociodemographic factors, not now incorporated into the AAPCC, could account for an additional 5 to 10 percent of costs (Thomas and Lichtenstein, 1986). Thus, even using relatively unsophisticated screening and selective marketing approaches, HMOs could attract a population with costs of 10 to 15 percent below average utilization. This would cost the Medicare program almost $1 billion in 1990 and close to $4 billion by the year 2000. For the most part, these costs will be avoided if HMOs marketing practices are standardized.

Savings from Prospective Physician Payment

We have too little experience to directly assess the impact of prospective pricing through a RVU scale on physician behavior. However, the past performance of prospective reimbursement for hospitals and nursing homes has been quite consistent. Relative to cost-based payments, PPSs lead to reduced escalation of costs, roughly equal to 3 percent of total costs per year (Eby and Cohodes, 1985). Assuming that the relative value scale has roughly comparable effects on physician pricing and utilization, a system initiated in 1990 would by the year 2000 lead to savings of roughly $4 billion annually.

The national cost targets recommended here would undoubtedly generate more efficient delivery of care and additional savings for the program. Because we have no way of estimating the extent of current unnecessary utilization of physician services and because we wish to make our predictions for savings conservative we have assumed here a very moderate limitation on growth of expenditures: about 7 percent per year. This generates roughly $1.5 billion in annual savings by 2000.

Savings from Hospital Payment Reforms

The proposed changes in hospital reimbursement may reduce costs in two ways. First, creating a budget constraint for each hospital will tend to cap utilization, capturing some of the same cost savings as does prepayment in HMOs. Second, prospective budgeting eliminates the added incentive for increasing costs now found in DRGs, the incentive to readmit patients a number of times to maximize revenues.

Prospective budgeting should eliminate some of the hospitalization that has traditionally made fee-for-service health care more expensive than that provided in prepaid settings. Because, however, fee-for-service hospitalization rates have recently fallen, the gap between fee-for-service and prepaid care has narrowed. It is impossible to determine how long and to what extent this trend will continue, but it seems likely that general Medicare hospitalization rates in the future will be on the order of 10 percent greater than in prepaid settings as opposed to the historical difference of between 20 and 30 percent. Assuming that prospective budgeting can capture only one-half this difference, it could induce cost reductions of roughly $2 billion to $4 billion annually. Additional savings might be realized if the budget caps are successful at reducing hospitalization rates to levels closer to those found in prepaid settings.

Savings created by eliminating the incentive for readmission are difficult to predict with any accuracy. Readmissions under the DRG system will be a problem only to the extent that hospitals (through physicians) are able to induce changes in the pattern of patient treatment. Any evidence of this effect has to this point been obscured by the large secular declines in hospital admission rates. Studies of other aspects of physician-induced demand, though, suggests that this effect will likely be small (Wilensky and Rossiter, 1983). Lacking better evidence, we predict that readmission might lead to perhaps a 2-to-3-percent increase in aggregate hospital costs, or $1.5 billion to $2 billion in the year 2000. Consequently, we predict savings of equal magnitude under our revised hospital payment system.

Costs of Uncompensated Care

Based on current estimates of the costs of free care and bad debt and assuming these costs remain proportional to total hospital expenditures, total hospital uncompensated care should approach $11 billion (in 1985 dollars) in the year 2000 (Oshfeldt, 1985). Medicare's share would slightly exceed $4 billion annually.

Costs Shifted by Requiring Uniform Medicaid Eligibility for Elderly

Requiring that all elders with incomes at or below 125 percent of the poverty line be covered by Medicaid would affect between 20 and 25 percent of all Medicare beneficiaries. This represents somewhat more than a doubling of the total fiscal obligations for the Medicaid program (U.S. Congress, Senate, Special Committee on Aging, 1984). Because, however, Medicaid is no longer responsible for paying for long-term care, the overall cost of the program will decline. States' expenditures are predicted to fall by roughly $4 billion yearly.

REFERENCES

Bishop, C. E. 1981. A Compulsory National Long-Term-Care Insurance Program. In *Reforming the Long-Term Care System*, ed. J. J. Callahan, Jr., and S. S. Wallack, pp. 61–93. Lexington, MA: D. C. Heath.

Cafferata. G. 1984. *Private Health Insurance Coverage of the Medicare Population: Data Preview 18.* U.S. Department of Health and Human Services, Public Health Service, Office of the Assistant Secretary for Health, National Center for Health Services Research.

Commonwealth of Massachusetts, Executive Office of Human Services. 1986. *Hospital Reimbursement and Access to Care: Chapter 372 and Beyond.* Pub. No. 14–423–243–300–4–86–C.R.

Eby, C., and D. Cohodes. 1985. What Do We Know About Rate Setting? *Journal of Health Politics, Policy and Law* 10 (2):299–313.

Eggars, P. W., and R. Prihoda. 1982. Pre-enrollment Reimbursement Patterns of Medicare Beneficiaries Enrolled in 'At-Risk' HMOs. *Health Care Financing Review* 4 (1):55–73.

Harvard Medicare Project. 1986. *Medicare: Coming of Age. A Proposal for Reform.* Boston: Division of Health Policy Research and Education, Harvard University.

Hicks, B., H. Raisz, J. Segal et al. 1981. The Triage Experiment in Coordinated Care for the Elderly. *American Journal of Public Health* 71 (9):991–1003.

Johnson,C. L., and L. A. Grant. 1985. *The Nursing Home in American Society.* Baltimore, MD: Johns Hopkins University Press.

Lifson, A. 1984. Long-Term Care: An Insurer's Perspective. In *Long-Term-Care Financing and Delivery Systems: Exploring Some Alternatives.* Washington: Health Care Financing Administration.

Long, S. H., R. F. Settle and C. R. Link. 1982. Who Bears the Burden of Medicare Cost Sharing? *Inquiry* 19 (3):222–34.

Manning, W. G., K. B. Wells and B. Benjamin. 1986. *Use of Outpatient Mental Health Care.* Rand Pub. No. R–3277–NIMH. Santa Monica, CA: Rand Corporation.

Manton, K. G., and K. Liu. 1984. *The Future Growth of the Long-Term Care Population: Projections Based on the 1977 National Nursing Home Survey and the 1982 Long-Term Care Survey.* Presented at the Third National Leadership Conference on Long-Term Care Issues, Washington, March 7–9.

Morris, R., and P. Youket. 1981. The Long-Term Care Issues: Identifying the Problems and Potential Solutions. In *Reforming the Long-Term Care System,* ed. J. J. Callahan, Jr., and S. S. Wallack, pp. 11–28. Lexington, MA: Lexington Books.

Oshfeldt, R. 1985. Uncompensated Medical Services Provided by Physicians and Hospitals. *Medical Care* 23 (12):1388–44.

Rice, D. P., and J. J. Feldman. 1983. Living Longer in the United States: Demographic Changes and Health Needs of the Elderly. *Milbank Memorial Fund Quarterly* 61 (3):362–96.

Russell, L. B. 1981. An Aging Population and the Use of Medical Care. *Medical Care* 19 (6):633–43.

Shapiro, S., E. A. Skinner, M. Kramer et al. 1985. Measuring Need for Mental Health Services in a General Population. *Medical Care* 23 (9):1033–43.

Sharfstein, S. S., S. Muszynski and E. Meyers. 1984. *Health Insurance and Psychiatric Care: Update and Appraisal.* Washington: American Psychiatric Press.

Soldo, B. J., and K. G. Manton. 1985. Changes in the Health Status and Service Needs of the Oldest Old: Current Patterns and Future Trends. *Milbank Memorial Fund Quarterly,* 63 (2):286–323.

Thomas, J., and R. Lichtenstein. 1986. Including Health Status in Medicare's Adjusted Average per Capita Cost Capitation Formula. *Medical Care* 24 (3):259–74.

U.S. Congress. House. Select Committee on Aging. 1985. *America's Elderly at Risk.*

U.S. Congress. Senate. Special Committee on Aging. 1984. *Medicare and the Health Costs of Older Americans: The Extent and Effects of Cost Sharing.* 98th Congress, 2d session.

U.S. Department of Health and Human Services. National Center for Health Statistics,

Public Health Service. 1985. *Health, United States 1985*. DHHS Pub. No. (PHS) 86–1232.

Waldo, D. R., and H. C. Lazenby. 1984. Demographic Characteristics and Health Care Use and Expenditures by the Aged in the United States: 1977–1984. *Health Care Financing Review* 6 (1):1–29.

Weissert, W. G. 1985. Estimating the Long-Term Care Population: Prevalence Rates and Selected Characteristics. *Health Care Financing Review* 6 (4):83–91.

Wilensky, G. R., and Louis F. Rossiter. 1983. The Relative Importance of Physician-Induced Demand in the Demand for Medical Care. *Milbank Memorial Fund Quarterly* 61 (2):252–77.

Authors and Participants in the Harvard Medicare Project

Nancy J. Altman is a lecturer in Public Policy, John F. Kennedy School of Government, Harvard University, and a Lecturer in Law at Harvard Law School. She is a lawyer with extensive experience in public policy legislation. Prior to coming to Harvard, she served as Executive Assistant to Dr. Alan Greenspan, Chairman of the National Commission on Social Security Reform; as Executive Assistant to the Undersecretary of the Department of Education, and as legislative assistant to Senator John C. Danforth of Missouri, where she had responsibilities in the areas of health and income maintenance.

Judith Bentkover is an Adjunct Lecturer of Public Policy at the Kennedy School of Government, Harvard University, and a Lecturer of Economics in the Department of Health Policy and Management at the Harvard School of Public Health. As Director of Policy Analysis and Special Projects at the Greater Boston Forum for Health Action, Inc., she recently supervised the planning of projects to promote the provision of affordable, high quality health care in the Greater Boston Area. Formerly Senior Health Economist and Manager of the Health Economics and Policy Unit at Arthur D. Little, Inc., Dr. Bentkover has extensive experience in the successful design and implementation of federal, state and local health care decision making as well as strategic planning for the private health care sector. Dr. Bentkover's publications include books and articles on health services research methods and health care policy analysis.

Robert Binstock is Henry R. Luce Professor of Aging, Health and Society in the Department of Epidemiology and Biostatistics at the School of Medicine, Case Western Reserve University. A former President of the Gerontological Society of America (1975–76), he has served as director of a White House Task Force on Older Americans in 1967–68, and as chairman and member of a number of advisory panels on aging to the U.S. government. He is currently a member of the National Academy of Sciences Committee on an Aging Society. Author of over 80 articles on politics and policies affecting aging, his seven books include: *Feasible Planning for Social Change, International Perspectives on Aging: Population and Policy Challenges*, and *Handbook of Aging and the Social Sciences.*

David Blumenthal was Executive Director of the Center for Health Policy, and Lecturer in Public Policy at the John F. Kennedy School of Government, Harvard University, until February, 1987. He is currently Senior Vice President of the Brigham and Women's Medical Center, Inc., in Boston. From 1977–79, Dr. Blumenthal was a professional staff member of the Senate Subcommittee on Health and Scientific Research, chaired by Senator Edward M. Kennedy. There he drafted legislation related to technology policy, the study of regulation of health maintenance organizations, and the provision of preventive health services and other matters. Dr. Blumenthal's research and writing concern federal policy toward health care technology, the comparative performance of for-profit and nonprofit health care systems, and university/industry relationships in biotechnology.

Philip Caper, an internist, is Professor of Community and Family Medicine at Dartmouth Medical School. Dr. Caper has also been the President of the Codman Research Group since 1984. He was the Chairman of the National Council on Health Planning and Development, the major standing federal advisory committee on matters of health policy from 1980–83, and a charter member of that Council from 1977–83. From 1976–80, prior to coming to Harvard, Dr. Caper was Vice Chancellor for Health Affairs and Professor of Medicine and of Community and Family Medicine at the University of Massachusetts Medical School. While there, he was chief of the medical staff and interim Director of the University Hospital. From 1971–76, he was a Professional Staff Member of the U.S. Senate Subcommittee on Health. He is the author of numerous papers on the financing and regulation of medical care.

Hale Champion was Executive Dean of the Kennedy School of Government, Harvard University until March 1987. He is currently Chief Secretary to the governor of Massachusetts, and was Undersecretary of the Department of Health, Education and Welfare from 1977–79. He has been a congressional aide, a vice president for finance at Harvard University and the University of Minnesota, Director of the Boston Redevelopment Authority, and Press Secretary, Executive Secretary, and Director of Finance for California's Governor Edmund G. Brown. He is a trustee of the National Academy of Public Administration; and a director of the National Center for Social Policy, (the Henry J. Kaiser Family Foundation), and the Multibank Financial Corporation.

Pamela Brown Drumheller was Coordinator of the Harvard Medicare Project at the Center for Health Policy and Management and, subsequently, Coordinator of Special Projects at the Institute for the Study of Smoking Behavior and Policy, both at the John F. Kennedy School of Government, Harvard University. She is currently Project Director at the Department of Maternal and Child Health, Harvard School of Public Health.

Rashi Fein, Professor of the Economics of Medicine at Harvard Medical School, is a former member of the Senior Staff of President Kennedy's Council of Economic Advisors. From 1963–68, he served as senior staff member of the Economic Studies Division of the Brookings Institution, Washington. He is the author/co-author of over 70 articles and five books in the field of medical care organization and financing, including *A Right to Health: The Problem of Access to Primary Care* (with Charles Lewis and David Mechanic), and, most recently, *Medical Care, Medical Costs: The Search for a Health Insurance Policy.*

William Hsiao, Professor of Economics and Health Policy at the Harvard School of Public Health, was Chief Actuary for Health Programs, U.S. Department of

Health, Education and Welfare. He has served as consultant to the Secretary of the Department of Health and Human Services, as well as to Congress on the financing of Medicare and Medicaid programs and the restructuring of the Social Security Program. He has also served as advisor to state government officials on health care facility planning and regulation of health care costs and insurance rates.

Theodore R. Marmor taught at the Universities of Wiconsin, Minnesota, and Chicago before coming to Yale in 1979 as Chairman for the Center for Health Studies. He is Professor of Public Management and Political Science at the Yale University School of Organization and Management and Department of Political Science. Professor Marmor is the author of *The Politics of Medicare*, *Political Analysis and American Medical Care*, and of numerous articles emphasizing social security, national health insurance and health planning. He was editor of the *Journal of Health Policy, Politics and Law* from 1980–84.

Alicia H. Munnell is Senior Vice President and Director of Research with the Federal Reserve Bank of Boston. Dr. Munnell has served as a member of the National Academy of Public Administration, the Institute of Medicine, the Pension Research Council for the Wharton School of Finance and Commerce, and the Associated Staff of the Brookings Institution, Washington. Her books include *The Economics of Private Pensions* and *The Future of Social Security*.

Julius B. Richmond, John D. MacArthur Professor of Health Policy and Management at the Kennedy School of Government and Professor of Health Policy at the Harvard Medical School and Harvard School of Public Health, is Director of the Division of Health Policy Research and Education at Harvard University. From 1977–81, he was Surgeon General of the United States Public Health Service, and Assistant Secretary for Health, U.S. Department of Health, Education and Welfare. The founder and former National Director of Project Head Start, Dr. Richmond also currently serves as a consultant to the Department of Psychiatry at Children's Hospital Medical Center, Boston, Massachusetts. Dr. Richmond also served as Professor and Chairman of the Department of Pediatrics and Dean of the Medical Faculty of the School of Medicine, State University of New York at Syracuse.

Mark Schlesinger is Assistant Director of the Center for Health and Human Resources Policy, Kennedy School of Government, Harvard University. His ongoing research interests include comparative studies of nonprofit and for-profit health care facilities, health policy issues affecting the elderly, and the relative roles of the market and government in the provision of health and social services. He is co-editor and an author of the forthcoming book, *Children in A Changing Health Care System.*

Joel I. Suldan served on the staff of the Harvard Medicare Project while he was a student at Harvard Law School, from which he graduated in 1985. He is currently an attorney specializing in health law with the Washington, D.C. office of the firm of McDermott, Will & Emery.

James M. Verdier is a Lecturer in Public Policy at the Kennedy School of Government, Harvard University, since 1983. He served for eight years in the Tax

Analysis Division of the U.S. Congressional Budget Office, heading the division from 1979–83. He authored three CBO publications on tax-policy issues, and supervised numerous others, including one on tax subsidies for medical care. Before coming to CBO, he served as a legislative assistant for Representative Henry S. Reuss (1968–72) and Senator Walter F. Mondale (1973–75).

Terrie Wetle Assistant Professor of Medicine, Harvard Medical School, is Associate Director of the Division on Aging, Harvard University. Formerly, she was Director of an area agency on aging in Oregon, and a social policy analyst for the Administration on Aging, Department of Health, Education and Welfare. She currently serves on the Geriatric Consult Team and Elder Abuse Assessment Team, Beth Israel Hospital, Boston, Massachusetts. From 1979–81, she was Director of the Program in Long Term Care, Yale University School of Medicine. Her books include *Handbook of Geriatric Care* and *Older Veterans: Linking VA and Community Resources*.

Index